Medical Malpractice Risk Management

Second Edition

by Vicente Franklin Colón, MD, James Scheper, JD, and Nicholas Bunch, JD

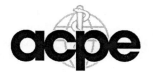

American College of Physician Executives
400 North Ashley Drive, Suite 400
Tampa, Florida 33602
813-287-2000

ISBN: 0-9787306-2-3

Library of Congress Card Number: 2011-907785

Printed in the United States of America by Lightning Source, Inc., St. Louis, MO.

Preface

For the past 50 years, physicians have been exposed to an ever-present and nagging fact: any patient may sue at any time for a disappointment or unfulfilled expectation. This fact of life has changed the character of medicine from what it was when I first began to practice medicine in the early 1960s. As medical practice has become more effective in reducing morbidity and mortality, the expectations of the public as to what is possible have become inflated. Some of those expectations are not without a rational basis, but expectations have sometimes gone beyond the realm of reality. Forty years ago, I heard a colleague quip that the expectations of the general public were so high that he expected to see a magazine article entitled "New Hope for the Dead" published somewhere in the popular literature.

Some feel that we may be closer to that situation than we might like to admit. Modern medical technology has allowed us to perform what some call miracles, but in our current economy miracles are not available to everyone. Some of our technologies seem to extend lives while actually prolonging the processes of death. The inability to return every treated patient to a full life and perfect health is interpreted by some to be a sign of negligence in the use of our miraculous technologies. The failure to provide miracles for everyone is considered a professional failure by some members of the public and even by some fellow professionals. In some cases, the disparity between professional reality and the expectations of the public can lead to litigation.

Over the years, many of us who have had a good deal of experience in dealing with malpractice litigation have formed our own opinions as to what are the most common causes of lawsuits. Most often the instigating problem lies in doctor-patient communication. One of the fathers of modern psychiatry, Alan Gregg, put his finger on it when he said that "more errors are made by those who do not care rather than those who do not know." Whereas technical failures are sometimes the cause of a malpractice claim, the more common precipitants of litigation by patients or their families are feelings of being ignored by the physician or by a lack of empathy.

Over my many years as a medical educator, I have been astounded by the fact that most medical colleges do not prepare medical students to deal with one of the pressing issues of medical practice in the USA. During my years as Professor of Family Medicine at the University of Cincinnati, I decided that I would spend a sabbatical year studying law. In the time that I had at the University of Cincinnati College of Law, I focused on learning as much about tort law and medical malpractice as I could. The law college was extremely generous and allowed me to take as many courses as I could fit in. I was granted the appellation, Scholar in Residence. That honor allowed me to take upper level as well as entrance level courses. I loaded my schedule and had the privilege of investigating, in depth, just what it was that went on that so terrified us physicians. What became clear to me was that the lawyers are given the responsibility for learning and enforcing the rules by which society functions. Their job is to make certain that the rights of individuals and of societal institutions are protected. On the other hand we as physicians generally do not have a clue as to what the rules of this game are, even though we play a very important role in the well-being of our society. As I learned more about the law, I decided that my fellow physicians needed a compact source of information that would instruct them in the basics of law and how to deal with legal issues if and when they were confronted by them. This book is the outcome of my concern for the educational needs of physicians as they relate to the law.

I initially began by designing a series of seminars for physicians in 1989. In those seminars it was my purpose to help physicians to gain confidence in dealing with legal issues through developing familiarity with the legal process. Second, I wanted to make medical students and physicians aware of just how medical malpractice claims arise. Third, I wanted them to understand that malpractice claims can be drastically reduced through a series of prudent medical practice assessment steps, and, last, I wanted to instruct them on how to behave to avoid litigation and, should it occur, how to behave professionally to minimize the chance of negative outcomes in the legal system.

Over 20 years ago I had the privilege of working with Reece and Dascha Pierce of American Medical Seminars. With their help the Malpractice Seminar Series was established in Sarasota, Florida, in 1989. I was fortunate to have the support of my good friends, James Scheper, Esq., and Nicholas Bunch, Esq., over the next 11 years. In those 11 years we refined the content of our presentations. In 2000 I dropped out as a presenter in the series but Nick Bunch decided to continue and found himself a top notch associate, James Triona, Esq. The seminars continue to this day. This book is the product of the over 20 years that we have spent teaching and answering the excellent questions of our physician students at these seminars. The seminars have been popular because of the fact that there is a need for physicians to attain basic legal knowledge and because my associates have the interests of physicians at heart. They understand that maintaining high medical standards protects physicians and patients alike. Together, we have written this book with the intent of decreasing legal risks to the physicians who read it and employ the suggestions presented.

The book is brief because, as a physician, I understand that most docs are not going to pick up a big book on law and medicine. This one can be read in a couple of sittings, and I'm certain that you will find the experience of benefit. A physician friend of mine called me a while back with these words, "I wish I had read your book before I got sued rather than after, as I did. It would have saved me a lot of trouble." Read on now and learn how to protect yourself, your associates and staff, and your family by learning the principals of *Medical Malpractice Risk Management*.

In this book we define *Medical Malpractice Risk Management* as the prudent practice of identifying and avoiding clinical and behavioral risks that can produce a significant negative impact on a physician's medical practice, and financial and personal well-being. The risks with which we are especially concerned pertain to damage to professional reputation, significant financial loss and the infliction of great personal emotional distress. Our objective is to provide the reader with enough insight into malpractice law to avoid falling into practice pitfalls that can create a risk of litigation.

Because this is a book on law, you knew that there had to be a disclaimer; so here it is. Because the statutes governing medical liability vary from state to state, I have to tell you that this book is written as a general guide to physicians and is not intended to provide specific legal advice. My colleagues and I strongly recommend that you have an attorney on retainer, even if you do not have current legal problems, to advise you of your rights and responsibilities should a circumstance that might trigger a malpractice action arise. It is imperative to seek immediate advice from an attorney well versed in the statutes governing medical liability in your specific jurisdiction. "Talk to your attorney before you talk to anyone else" is good advice. Having someone whom you can trust to give you good legal advice, should a problem come up, will save you a lot of stress and behavioral errors.

Vicente Franklin Colón, MD
March 2011

Introduction

Do concerns about medical malpractice cause you to lose sleep? If they do, you have opened the right book.

This book has been written by a physician with the assistance and guidance of two very experienced trial lawyers whose specialty is medical malpractice litigation. One of the attorneys is a well-respected defense lawyer and the other a highly respected plaintiff's attorney. Our common objective in writing this book is to help physicians and others interested in health care to acquire an understanding of the basics of the legal process; how to survive a medical malpractice claim, should it arise; and how to minimize its effects on a potential defendant through prudent planning and practice. When you have finished this book, you will:

- Have a sense of the legal parameters and the legal theories and issues that pertain to medical malpractice litigation and ways to protect your practice, your colleagues and you through prudent planning and preventive measures.

- Understand the concepts of standard of care, deviations from the standard, proximate cause, and damages.

- Recognize and understand how to assist your attorney in effective defense strategies.

- Be familiar with the various elements of a developing suit, such as the complaint and answer, discovery, expert witness, and trial procedures.

- Have an understanding of how various parties to a lawsuit relate to one another and should behave. It is important not to lose one's case because of inappropriate or unprofessional behavior.

You will have the fundamental knowledge to develop an effective, personalized risk management strategy structured to prevent or, at least, significantly reduce medical malpractice exposure.

Physicians See Themselves as Victims of an Unfair and Arbitrary Legal System

Medical malpractice is a term that sends shivers up and down the spines of many strong and hardy physicians. Mention the term in a medical staff lounge and one will hear more gnashing of teeth and cries of despair than there are in the entire biblical book of Lamentations. The reason otherwise self-assured, competent professionals are so intimidated by the idea of being sued by a disgruntled patient is that they see themselves as victims of a system that is unfair and arbitrary. Many physicians feel that they are committed to the care and well-being of patients who, at any moment, may decide to bite the hand that comforts them. That sometimes is true, but it is our experience that physicians are more likely to feel themselves to be potential victims of malpractice litigation because they do not understand the societal and legal rules surrounding the practice of medicine and have no useful preventive strategies to deal with the legal risks inherent in their work.

Personal Education Regarding Malpractice Pitfalls Will Reduce Anxiety as Well as Risks of Medical Malpractice Litigation

The authors of this book have spent more than 20 years devising seminar curricula to help physicians understand the basic elements of medical malpractice law. It has been our principal objective to demonstrate to physicians that they are not powerless in the legal milieu. Physicians have a great many opportunities to minimize legal risks by developing an understanding of the rules of the medicolegal game that are encompassed in tort law. Tort law is the part of the civil law that allows for monetary compensation of a party injured by the negligence of another. Understanding tort law is basic to developing effective risk management strategies. Attendees of the seminars that we have presented over the years have expressed to us a sense of empowerment as they gained an understanding of how the legal process works and how each physician is able to tailor his or her practice activities to minimize exposure to liability.

Physicians Need to Accept the Fact that the Law Views Medical Care as a Service Commodity

It is essential that every physician, just as every category of business person, understand the special responsibilities that he or she has in regard to services rendered to each patient or customer. Centuries-old rules of law and custom specify the duties of each party in a transaction, whether it is medical or commercial. Civil laws have been formulated over the centuries to support civilized behavior among parties involved in all types of transactions. It just so happens that, in medicine, the transaction between physician and patient involves the most precious of commodities—health and life itself. That makes the relationship particularly intimate and, at the same time, fragile. Other business persons have relationships with their customers, but they rarely have the special significance of the relationship between patient and physician. The duties of a paint vendor, for instance, are relatively mundane and focus principally on the quality of the product sold. On the other hand, the duties of the physician are very personal and extend from spiritual and psychological counseling to physical and pharmaceutical therapies. The patient-physician relationship is more intimate than almost any other non-family relationship and thus is subject to many of the same stresses that affect family relations.

The Cost of Doing Business

Both the business person and the physician need to understand that, no matter their intent, there will be problems with unhappy customers or patients. From time to time, both physicians and business people experience poor results despite their best efforts. Poor results can occur without there being any negligence, but there are times when lack of attention to detail and bad luck lead to unfortunate but avoidable outcomes. In these cases, customers/patients may seek legal recourse against a vendor or physician. Physicians must be prepared to deal with this type of uncomfortable event and for acrimony that an ordinary vendor does not normally receive. Unfortunately, in a doctor/patient relationship, there may be deep feelings of resentment when things do not go as planned, because of the very personal mature of the relationship. We want to emphasize to the reader that customer dissatisfaction is what the proprietor of any business must consider as one of the costs of doing business. Malpractice insurance is also a cost of doing business, as is the seemingly endless paperwork necessary for thoroughly recording interactions with patients, tests, and treatments. Every element of medical practice that protects the patient and enhances the quality of care is a cost of doing business. Physicians need to realize that the law sees medical practice as a part of commerce and not as a healing art separate in nature from other forms of commerce. If that becomes a part of the thinking of physicians, legal risks will induce less anxiety and less intense personal recriminations.

Physicians Take Legal Actions Very Personally, Frequently to Their Detriment

Physicians are often emotionally devastated by lawsuits. The qualities that make a good physician also make personal pain in malpractice litigation very likely. In many cases, physicians internalize the fact that they are being sued and feel themselves to be incompetent failures. They view the process of litigation not only as an unjust interference in what they do best, patient care, but also as a personal assault on their integrity and reputations. Anxiety, guilt, and depression, along with a sense of victimization, are common and extremely debilitating to many physicians ensnared in malpractice litigation. Anger and vengeance are often expressed, emotions that act to the detriment of the physician, his family, and patients. If the physician can accept the fact that legal liability exposure is *a cost of doing business*, these emotions, although still present, will not be as emotionally injurious as they are in the individual who takes the process personally and feels totally vulnerable.

Patients Sue Their Physicians for a Variety of Reasons

A legal truism is that no one is immune from the threat of lawsuits. There is no doubt that there are patients who maliciously sue physicians for a variety of perverse reasons. Others sue for nuisance purposes to try to wring a few dollars out of the system, but most patients who become plaintiffs truly believe that they have been injured through the negligence of caregivers. They often do not grasp the technical facts of the matter, but they do know that their expectations were not met in some way that was very important to them. Anger is a product of unmet expectations. Some sue without malice toward their physicians, but see a suit as a way to justify their own behaviors and to shift blame. We strongly encourage physicians to try to be as objective as possible in their personal and emotional responses to such events. Calm and prudent behavior in response to a claim of medical error preserves dignity and helps in the process of planning an effective response strategy.

Lawyers on Both Sides Have a Societal Responsibility to Seek Out Truth

Plaintiff lawyers are not, as a whole, the soulless scum that they are so often portrayed to be in medical lounges. They are frequently intelligent and committed individuals whose social responsibility is to provide the best possible representation to their clients. It is also the case that some do occasionally file poorly thought out, unmeritorious suits for their clients. Let us not deny, however, that physicians do make patient care errors, and there are valid claims made against them. On the other hand, defense lawyers are not always paragons of virtue, although most are intelligent, competent and ethical. The legal process is designed to find the truth of a matter, and attorneys on both sides play large roles in making certain that this usually happens. We urge our readers to treat attorneys on both sides of a suit with respect and courtesy, not only because it makes the process much less onerous but also because attorneys strive to fulfill a very important duty that society has placed on them, to protect the rights of us all.

The Majority of Medical Malpractice Claims Evolve in Favor of Physicians

Most malpractice claims do not make it to a jury, or even to court. Insurance company statistics reveal that only about 10 percent of the cases that come to their attention as possible malpractice claims are ever filed with a court. Of the 10 percent brought to court, 80 to 90 percent are either dismissed or have jury verdicts in favor of the defendant physician. The law places a heavy burden on plaintiffs to prove that physicians have, through acts of commission or omission, injured them and that they deserve to receive compensation for those errors. It is true that, in the past three decades, the number of lawsuits filed has increased and awards have risen, but the sensational press has made the situation appear worse than it really has been. Some legal experts claim that the medical malpractice insurance carriers also have an interest in keeping the pot stirred.

Asset Protection

There is such a thing as a poor outcome even when every effort has been made in a clinical effort on behalf of a patient. It is also a fact that even competent physicians and other caregivers make unfortunate errors that might cause a preventable patient injury. Although these are unintentional errors of judgment or skill, they nonetheless culminate in injury, pain, and suffering. Tort law governs these circumstances in our society and allows for the compensation of medical malpractice victims monetarily rather than through criminal penalties. The intent of tort law is to make the injured party "whole," i.e., return the injured person to the condition they enjoyed in life prior to the injury rather than inflict criminal punishments on the tortfeasor, the person who inflicted the injury. That is a big step up from the Code of Hammurabi, where the physician, more or less, had the same type injury inflicted upon him as the one caused. Economic compensation, which is at the heart of tort law, makes it essential that physicians adequately insure themselves against liability risks in order to protect their livelihoods, their personal assets, and the well-being of their families. It is also wise to incorporate into a personal economic plan life and personal liability insurance as well as appropriate estate planning. This is best done with the help of a well-qualified estate attorney.

In summary, this book is designed to be easy to read, it is not intended to be a comprehensive textbook on medical malpractice. We have laid out the most common issues that lead to medical malpractice suits in a simple, understandable format. Because state laws differ, the descriptions in this handbook may not fit every situation, but they will be useful in providing a general understanding of the legal principles that govern malpractice law. Whenever there is a question regarding the legal issues related to your practice, we encourage you to consult with a respected attorney who is well-versed in the malpractice laws of your state. On the other hand, the laws of most states are similar in intent. They provide a legal pathway for an injured party (the plaintiff) to claim damages (monetary compensation) from the party or parties responsible for an injury (the defendant(s)). This book will provide you with a basic understanding of where the pitfalls are and of safe pathways to follow to negotiate the medical malpractice maze.

Having a malpractice defense attorney on retainer for quick legal advice should a legal issue appear is a very prudent thing to do. The advice of a personal attorney can minimize and perhaps avoid many of the problems that emotionally upset physicians tend to get themselves into when a legal threat arises. Legal advice from a personal lawyer is privileged and provides experienced direction on legal processes and on personal behavior. It is an excellent expenditure.

About the Authors

Vicente Franklin Colón, MD, is Emeritus Professor of Family Medicine, University of Cincinnati College of Medicine; Director Emeritus and founder of the Bethesda Family Practice Residency Program, Cincinnati, Ohio, and Originator, Seminars on Medical Malpractice for the American Medical Seminars of Sarasota Florida.

Dr. Colón earned his undergraduate degree from Nebraska Wesleyan University and his medical degree from the University of Nebraska College of Medicine. He served his internship at Bryan Memorial Hospital, Lincoln, Nebraska, and initiated the mini-residency programs in anesthesiology and obstetrics/gynecology at the University of Nebraska.

Dr. Colón has authored and co-authored an extensive list of articles published in a wide variety of clinical journals as well as several medical textbook chapters and co-wrote a text book on clinical cytology. He has been a frequent speaker at conferences on medicolegal issues and has served on various medical association and governmental committees as well as task forces dealing with liability and risk management topics.

Dr. Colón is a life member of the American Medical Association and the American Academy of Family Physicians. He has been an officer in the Ohio Academy of Family Physicians and a member in the Society of Teachers of Family Medicine and the American College of Physician Executives. He was named Medical Educator of the Year in 1998 by the Ohio Academy of Family Physicians.

James H. Scheper, JD, is a partner with Shea & Associates, a Cincinnati law firm. He has been admitted to the bars of Ohio and California and to the U.S. District Court, Southern District of Ohio; the U.S. 6th District Court of Appeals; and the U.S. Supreme Court.

Mr. Scheper received his undergraduate education at Xavier University in Cincinnati and his law degree from the Salmon P. Chase College of Law at Northern Kentucky University. He is a member of the American Board of Trial Advocates, the Butler County Trial Lawyers Association, and the Butler County Mediation Board. He is a frequent speaker and faculty member at conferences and seminars on medicolegal topics.

Nicholas E. Bunch, JD, is a partner with the Cincinnati-based law firm White, Getgey & Meyer. He has been admitted to the bar of Ohio and to the United States District Court, Southern District of Ohio; the United States Tax Court; and the United States Court of Claims. He is a member of the bar associations of Ohio, Cincinnati, and Butler County.

Mr. Bunch received his undergraduate education at Ohio State University and his law degree from the University of Dayton School of Law. He is a member of the Ohio Academy of Trial Lawyers and the Hamilton County Trial Lawyers Association. He is a member of the

Negligence Law Committee of the Ohio State Bar Association. He is also a member of the Institutional Review Board of the University of Cincinnati College of Medicine.

Both Mr. Scheper and Mr. Bunch are experienced medical malpractice trial lawyers.

Acknowledgments

The authors want to thank those patient ladies whom we are fortunate enough to call our wives; Kathy Bunch, Joyce Scheper, and Marjorie Colón. Their support during our efforts in writing this book made it possible for us to spend hours discussing the structure of the book, writing it, and doing preliminary editing. To you ladies, we raise our glasses in a toast: Thank you so much.

We also want to thank our good friends Reece and Dascha Pierce of the American Medical Seminars, who provided us the opportunity to do our presentations on medical risk management for more than 20 years. It was in those seminars that the ideas for this book evolved. It is our hope that this book will serve to provide our readers a sense of comfort in their daily practice activities and to decrease the likelihood of the anguish that so many physicians experience when they become the defendants in a medical negligence suit.

Our gratitude also extends to the staff of the American College of Physician Executives, who have encouraged and helped us to make this book as easy to read as possible. The gentle direction has been much appreciated.

Contents

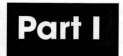

Part I

The Origins of
Medical Malpractice

Basic Elements of the Legal Process

Justice

"Justice is the earnest and constant will to render every man his due. The precepts of the law are these: to live honorably, to injure no other man, to render every man his due." Justinian I, the Byzantine emperor of the Sixth Century, captured the fundamental concept of law to which, even today, we hold fast. Justice is what we seek from God and our system of laws, but experience has taught us that justice is not as certain as we would like it to be.

The public has the right, and should make every effort, to know what goes on in its legal centers, but common news sources are not well geared to providing an accurate and balanced picture of many of the proceedings. Physicians are a part of that general public that is all too often confused about what actually goes on in our legal system. It behooves all of us to be just a little suspicious and critical of the headlines pertaining to trials that we read about or see in the media. We encourage anyone interested in learning more about the legal process to attend a high-profile trial and then read about it in the paper or listen to its description on television or radio. It immediately becomes evident that what happens and what is reported are often two different things.

Below we outline many issues in laws that pertain to physicians. Few physicians have familiarity with society's rules of the game as they pertain to medical practice. In this book there is the opportunity to become considerably more familiar with the salient issues. This book is considerably shorter than most books on Law and Medicine. It was written to entice physicians to learn how to defend themselves from suits and anxiety. This book is a relatively quick read; two to three hours. It is dedicated to physicians interested in minimizing the risks of becoming the object of medical malpractice action through basic understanding of legal principals and good in office and hospital medical practices.

Laws Are the Rules of Society

Laws are, in essence, the rules of the societal game, yet few understand the scope of law or its broad influence on everyday activities. Laws are first written broadly to restrict or enforce behaviors. They begin with general concepts and concerns in mind and are inevitably more narrowly interpreted as specific issues, falling within their purview, are examined. It's similar to the rules of golf. How many hackers have a clear idea of the options that a player has in dealing with a lateral water hazard? Few, and the misinterpretations and arguments are many. So the greatest problem in understanding legal process is not knowing or understanding the rules.

The Roles of Lawyers and Doctors

Society's specialists in the rules of everyday affairs are attorneys, and because the rules are so complex and are constantly being reworked via common law as well as legislation, they have to work hard to keep up with and mold these laws to their clients' benefit. Lawyers have a very heavy societal responsibility placed on them—preserving the rights of their clients. That's a considerably different societal burden from that placed on physicians, which is the health care of those same clients.

Lawyers are advocates for their clients. Their societal mission is clear and simple. They are to do everything, within the rules of law, to win for their side while discrediting the case of the other side. This is what the adversarial system is about. At one time, it was trial by combat to the death; now it's trial by word, ad nauseum.

In order to keep laws from becoming a jumble and the rule of force from becoming the mode, laws are organized into categories. Examples are criminal and civil law. Within those categories, procedural regulations have been established to allow each party in a legal fray to fairly present its side of the contested issues. The rules of procedure constitute another area of arcane knowledge. These rules deal with complaints, pleadings, trial procedures, evidence, and appeals. Each of those topics can be further broken down into subcategories. It is little wonder that the legal process is so poorly understood by lay people.

A Slow and Deliberate Process

In order to try to provide justice, the legal process is very slow and deliberate. Despite the clear-cut solutions so often depicted on television court shows, most legal actions are not resolved by a stroke of legal brilliance. They are carefully deliberated by a group of common people, our peers, who are educated on the facts of the case by each side of the litigated issues. Juries are the hearers of fact and must sort out the issues in the case at hand. Juries are usually, but not always, conscientious and resourceful. Even in complex cases, it is surprising how often they muddle through to an appropriate decision.

It generally takes a year or more from the filing of a lawsuit for a medical malpractice case to be fully prepared for trial. Medical records must be obtained and reviewed; medical literature supporting the opposing positions must be fully researched and understood; witnesses—both lay and expert—must be deposed. Often, there are legal issues that must be briefed and decided by the Court, each of which may have a significant impact on the outcome of the case.

Even a relatively "simple" medical malpractice case can take five or more days for the actual trial. The more complex the issues are, or the more defendants there are (each with a lawyer), the longer the trial process will be. Two-to-three-week-long trials are not beyond the norm.

Judges and Juries

Both plaintiffs and defendants are entitled to have a jury hear and decide the case. If both sides waive a jury trial, the case can be heard and decided, solely, by a judge. This is referred to as a "bench trial." This is unusual in medical malpractice cases, as each side typically perceives that their side of the case has particular appeal to a jury. Sympathy for the plaintiff and respect for the medical profession are just two reasons why parties often prefer trial by jury.

In jury trials, the judge and jury have separate and distinct roles. The judge presides over the legal issues in the proceedings, makes decisions about the testimony and the witnesses that will be presented to the jury, and provides the jury with instructions of the law applicable to the case just prior to the jury adjourning to consider its verdict. When a jury is empanelled, the judge does not decide the case. It is the jury's responsibility to consider all of the conflicting evidence that it has heard and decide the "facts" of the case. The jury will ultimately decide whether the evidence supports a finding that the standard of care was violated and resulted in injury to the patient. If it finds for the plaintiff, it then decides on the amount of money that will serve as reasonable compensation to the plaintiff. If the jury is persuaded that there was no deviation from the standard of care, or that, even if there was, the deviation did not cause injury to the patient; the jury will return a verdict in favor of the defendant.

Torts

Concepts and Elements

One of the most frequently and passionately debated issues over the past several years has been "tort reform." Almost everyone has an opinion on the matter, one that is often the result of personal experiences or shaped by widely circulated media accounts of "frivolous lawsuits," excessive awards, or unfair jury verdicts. To understand why this issue engenders such fervent discussion, it may be useful to review the evolution of the "tort system" and then focus on the development of medical malpractice cases in particular.

The word "tort" derives from the Latin "tortus," meaning "twisted." Under the French and English legal systems, the term has evolved to connote a *civil wrong* done in violation of another's rights. The legal definition of a tort is, "a civil wrong, other than a breach of contract, for which a court will provide a remedy in the form of equity damages." A tort is differentiated from a criminal wrong in the sense that the wrongdoer is not accused of violating a criminal statute and does not face criminal penalties such as fines or imprisonment. This is not to say, however, that criminal conduct cannot at times become the basis for a tort action. Indeed, many tort cases arise out of criminal conduct—assault, false imprisonment, driving under the influence of alcohol. These charges encompass elements of negligence that fall under the tort laws. A wrongdoer may well face a criminal prosecutor and then a civil proceeding for damages involving the same conduct. O. J. Simpson's criminal acquittal, which was followed by a large civil verdict against him, is a prime example.

A common theme that runs throughout the law of torts is that the liability of the wrongdoer, the "tortfeasor," is premised on an unreasonable interference with the rights and interests of others. Tort law deals with conduct that is socially unacceptable, and, if it produces harm to another, the tortfeasor will be held responsible for the damages. Many judicial critics have suggested that the field of tort law is a form of social engineering, in the sense that courts and juries determine what society deems to be acceptable or unacceptable behavior. Society has an inherent interest in deterring unreasonable behavior and in protecting the personal right to be free from injury caused by the negligent conduct of others.

The notion of victims seeking monetary compensation from tortfeasors can be traced to medieval England. Courts were originally interested only in keeping the "King's peace" and were not concerned with civil wrongs. Slowly, the courts came to appreciate that a breach of the King's peace might also involve a substantial loss to a royal subject and that compensation to the injured party was required to achieve true justice. For example, a teamster who negligently drove a team of horses through the crowded streets of a village without regard for pedestrians most assuredly broke the King's peace by inciting public panic. Additionally, if a villager sustained a broken leg from being struck by the horses, the teamster was required to compensate the victim for his inability to work.

Elements of a Tort Claim

When English courts decided cases, the decisions became part of the "common law." These legal decisions were then cited as precedents in other cases. This recognition of legal precedents in other courts added a certain uniformity and predictability to the resolution of disputes between parties. By the early 19th Century, the common law had developed four concepts essential to a successful tort claim. Those concepts remain ingrained in our system today. To prevail in a claim, the plaintiff must establish that:

- The defendant owed a *duty* of care to the plaintiff.

- The duty was *breached*.

- The breach *proximately (directly) caused injury* to the plaintiff.

- Damages were suffered by the plaintiff.

Failure to prove any one of these elements is fatal to a tort claim.

Duty

When we speak of "duty" in the context of the tort system, we are referring to an obligation for a person to conform to a certain standard of civil conduct. That standard is established and enforced for the protection of others against unreasonable risks. This duty of care obviously varies with each situation, but courts have generally held that the duty of care is premised on the foreseeability of harm that might result as a consequence of a person's acting, or not acting, in a certain manner; in essence, the greater the foreseeability of harm to others or their properties because of a particular action, the greater the likelihood that a duty of care will be *imposed on the actor*.

For example, laws that regulate speed limits on our streets involve an assessment of the foreseeability of the risk of harm. A driver is under a duty to drive 20 mph in a school zone because it is reasonably foreseeable that children may, unexpectedly, run into the street and that the posted slower speed can prevent injury. On the other hand, drivers on the expressway are allowed to drive 65 mph; it is highly unlikely that pedestrians will be darting into the flow of traffic.

Additionally, a relationship between one person and another can give rise to certain duties of care. For example, a business owner has the duty to maintain his premises in a reasonably safe condition for the protection of his patrons. A physician has the duty to provide patients a level of care that is recognized by other physicians to be within the range of accepted medical practice. On the other hand, the absence of a relationship between parties obviates any duty. A landowner has no relationship with a trespasser on his land and therefore has no duty to maintain his property in a reasonably safe condition for the trespasser. (Here is an Ohio Supreme Court case discussing the duties owed to a trespasser, "a landowner owes no duty to licensee or trespasser except to refrain from willful, wanton or reckless conduct which is likely to injure him." The duty owed by a landowner if he is aware that a trespasser, on his property, is in a position of peril is "to use ordinary care to avoid injury to him.") Likewise, it is generally held that a physician has no duty of care to anyone until a physician/patient relationship is established.

All civil conduct is measured by what is known as the "reasonable man" standard. The intent of this standard is to utilize objective criteria to measure behavior rather than to use purely subjective assessments of actions and consequences. The legal analysis is based on what a "reasonable person would do under the same or similar circumstances," rather than on what the actor (defendant) thought would be appropriate conduct. In medicolegal questions, a physician has a duty to patients to act as any physician of ordinary skill, care, and diligence would under the same or similar circumstances. Notice that the duty *does not require* the physician to act as the pre-eminent or most skillful practitioner would; rather, the duty is to act as a reasonable or ordinary physician would act. This is a special example of the "reasonable man" standard.

Whether a duty actually exists is usually a question of law for the judge to decide. In medicolegal cases, judges typically instruct jurors that the existence of a physician-patient relationship imposes upon the physician the obligation to provide medical care consistent with the accepted standard of care. Exactly what the "duty" consists of, in any given case, requires the testimony of medical experts, as jurors are not generally familiar with what physicians are expected to do in various medical situations. Each side to the case will present testimony from expert witnesses. These experts are usually doctors with points of view diametrically opposed to each other as to what exactly should have been done by the defendant. Juries are not charged with the question of whether a defendant owes a plaintiff a duty, but they must decide on the scope of duty in order to decide whether there was a breach of duty.

Breach of Duty

Once a duty of care has been established, the next inquiry is whether that duty was breached. A breach occurs when one fails to act as a "reasonable man" would act. If a person is acting as any other reasonably prudent person would act in a similar situation, there is no "breach of duty," even if the conduct produces an injury to another. For example, a driver who is traveling at the speed limit and is keeping a careful lookout will not be liable if he were to strike a child who suddenly darts out from behind a parked car. There was simply no breach of the driver's duty because he was driving in a careful and prudent manner.

If a person breaches the duty of care owed to another, he has, by law, acted negligently. He has neglected the societal obligation to act with due care. The objective reasonable man standard is applied in court to determine if, in fact, negligence has occurred. Foreseeability is pivotal to this determination.

With physicians, a breach of duty is often referred to as "a deviation from the accepted standards of care." This concept holds that a physician who fails to act as a reasonably prudent and skillful physician has fallen below the standard expected in a given situation. A family medicine practitioner is expected to review, understand, and take appropriate action regarding the results of any diagnostic tests ordered. Failure to do so constitutes a breach of his duty.

Just as proof of a physician's duty is established through the expert testimony of other physicians, so too the breach of that duty must also be proven by expert testimony. Any expert witness who seeks to criticize or defend the actions of a physician must be clearly aware of what is expected of a physician under the same or similar circumstances and then contrast the specific conduct of the physician in question with that standard. If a physician has failed to act in accordance with the profession's recognized methods of diagnosis and treatment, it is easy to argue that there has been a breach of duty.

Despite the enormous technical advances in the medical field, medicine remains as much an art as it is a science. The physician's ability to gather, organize, and comprehend information relating to a patient still involves a great deal of individual judgment and discretion. It is also true that there is often more than one acceptable method of assessment and treatment for a patient's condition. For example, there are diverse views on whether surgery or conservative management for certain spinal conditions yields a better result. For this reason, the law generally recognizes that, even if there is an untoward result in outcome, the physician has not breached his duty as long as he acted in accordance with the generally accepted and recognized method of treatment. Methods of treatment that are generally recognized by other responsible practitioners as being appropriate, discussed in the medical literature, discussed at medical conferences, and/or taught at medical schools are generally considered to be in accord with the "standard of care"; this constitutes evidence of no deviation from the standard of care. One must bear in mind that a bad outcome does not constitute negligence or bad medical practice.

Proximate Cause

A breach of duty does not always result in injury. Running a red light at 3:00 a.m. when there is no one in the crosswalk is a breach of the duty to obey traffic laws, but if no one is present to be injured, the breach cannot "proximately cause" an injury. The direct and natural relationship between an act and an injury is the linchpin of the concept of *proximate cause*. It satisfies a cause and effect analysis.

Proximate cause is said to exist when an act of omission or commission, in a natural and foreseeable continuous sequence of events, produces an injury. In addition, conditions must be such that without that purported act the injury would not have occurred. This is referred to as the "but for" test; the injury would not have occurred "but for" the action(s) of the tortfeasor. The limitation on the test is that the act must naturally, foreseeably, and continuously lead to the injury. An actor is not responsible for remote consequences of actions; remote is defined as a result that could not have been reasonably foreseen or anticipated. A negligent act must naturally and directly lead to an injury before the actor can be held liable for damages.

Establishing a proximate causal relationship between a physician's alleged negligent treatment and a patient's injury or death is the most difficult burden a plaintiff faces in medical malpractice cases. Indeed, many skilled defense lawyers concede the issue of deviation from the standard of care, but nonetheless mount a vigorous defense due to a lack of "proximate cause" between the negligence and the patient's injury or death. For example, it may be negligent for an obstetrician/gynecologist not to follow-up on a suspicious breast lump when it is first brought to his attention. If, two months later, another physician biopsies the mass and discovers cancer, a strong proximate cause defense can be asserted. It can be argued that the negligent delay in diagnosis caused by the first physician did not proximately cause any damage to the patient, because a two-month delay is not sufficient to change the patient's condition, treatment, or outcome significantly.

Similarly, a family practitioner who fails to diagnose a brain lesion might be faulted for failing to have ordered a CT scan or MRI of the head, but if the patient dies of an unsuspected MI the following week, it could be safely argued that any negligence on the part of the physician did not directly result in the patient's death. On the other hand, if a physician fails to heed a radiologist's recommendation for follow-up on an uncalcified lesion in the lung seen on a plain chest film, it is likely that a court will allow a claim to be made that asserts that the failure was the proximate cause of the patient's death from lung cancer three years later.

The more direct, reasonable and logical the link between an act and an injury, the higher the likelihood that proximate cause will be found. Frequently, jurors, in responses to written questions submitted to them following a malpractice trial, have commented that, even though they felt that the defendant deviated from the standard of care, the deviation did not cause the plaintiff's injuries. This is a critical and pivotal issue in medical negligence cases, so it often consumes the bulk of the testimony in a courtroom trial.

Damages

The plaintiff's final burden in a tort case is to prove the nature and extent of injuries proximately caused by the defendant's negligent act. The determination of damages is a direct extension of the proof of causation and points directly to the economic and other compensable consequences to the plaintiff from the injury sustained.

As an example, a plaintiff may demonstrate that a defendant's negligence, failing to yield the right-of-way, resulted in an intersection collision in which the plaintiff sustained a comminuted fracture of an ankle. Thus, the plaintiff has to prove that there was a natural and foreseeable relationship between the negligent act and a physical injury. To receive full compensation for the injury, the specific monetary consequences of the injuries must be demonstrated. Typically, the plaintiff includes past and future medical expenses, past and future lost income, impairments in the major activities of daily activities, and pain and suffering associated with the physical injury. In order to recover these damages, the plaintiff must prove that each loss is directly and naturally related to the negligence of the defendant. Certainly, a defendant may challenge the extent of past or future damages and is often assisted in this endeavor when the jury believes a plaintiff is exaggerating the injuries.

Our civil legal system is based on the premise that the proper method of compensation to an injured plaintiff is through a monetary award. In tort law there is no "eye for an eye." While monetary compensation seems well suited to damages such as medical expenses and lost income, it is problematic in other "damages" areas. What is it "reasonably" worth to endure the pain of a broken leg or a shattered ankle? What should a reasonable award be for a 35-year-old man who is permanently confined to a wheelchair? The most difficult kind of question, what amount of money should be awarded to fairly and reasonably compensate a 40-year-old widow with three children for the wrongful death of her husband? These are the issues that juries face in courthouses throughout this country.

Intentional Torts/Punitive Damages

The law distinguishes between negligent conduct that is unintentional and conduct that is intentional. In the latter situation, an actor, the defendant, has neglected to act with due care, carelessly and imprudently. In an *intentional tort* the actor recklessly and/or indifferently causes certain negative consequences. There is knowledge that given outcomes are substantially certain to result from the wrongful act or acts. In tort law intentional misconduct is punishable by awarding plaintiff punitive damages. Punitive damages are designed to punish a defendant and to deter others, by example, from engaging in similar conduct. It is important to know that most liability insurance policies exclude from coverage damages caused by the intentional acts of the insured. Medical malpractice cases rarely involve intentional misconduct, but when they do, the defendant cannot fall back on insurance coverage. In addition they are not tax deductible, nor is debt relief granted in bankruptcy.

Vicarious Liability

While the law usually focuses on the conduct of a specific actor in a tort, there are situations in which one may be held liable for damages caused by the actions of others. This is known as *vicarious liability* and is premised on the relationship between the actual tortfeasor and the one against whom damages are sought. Employer/employee, principal/agent, and master/servant relationships are the ones most commonly cited. These relationships involve the right of the person able to control the actions of the other individuals named in a suit. If an employer dispatches an employee to drive a company truck and the employee causes an accident, both the employee and employer are held liable. Hospitals are responsible for the negligent acts of employees such as paid medical staff, residents, nurses, and others.

Joint Tortfeasors

The law acknowledges that a single injury can be caused by the negligence of more than one person. Historically, an injured person was permitted to collect damages from any one or all of the defendants under the concept of *joint and several liability*. This concept is premised on the idea that if the wrongdoing of two or more persons causes indivisible injury, i.e., the plaintiff cannot attribute specific responsibility to any one of the defendants for the extent of an injury or injuries, each tortfeasor should be responsible for the entire damage. If one defendant paid more than his proportionate share of damages, he had the right to collect from other defendants for any payments in excess of his fair share of the award to the plaintiff.

Recently, states have enacted laws that limit any given defendant's liability to the specific percentage of fault in causing the injury, thus ending the notion that tortfeasors are "jointly" responsible for all damages. The newer laws focus on holding each person accountable for an amount commensurate with his individual conduct.

Comparative Fault

The law is in place to find truth and to work impartially. The law recognizes that people may actually contribute to their own injuries through their own contributory negligence. In the past, under most state laws, a plaintiff was denied any amount of recovery if found to be even the slightest bit at fault for causing or contributing to his injuries. Most jurisdictions came to view this "all or nothing" approach as too harsh and have enacted some variety of the "comparative fault" principle. Under this system, relative degrees of fault between plaintiff and defendant are determined by a jury. A plaintiff may recover only that percentage of the total damages that is attributed to the defendant(s). For example, in a case involving an anaphylactic reaction to penicillin, if a jury decides that the patient is 30 percent at fault for failing to provide accurate information on a medical history regarding penicillin sensitivity, but determines that the physician is 70 percent at fault for not eliciting an adequate history at the time of penicillin administration, the patient may recover 70 percent of damages caused by the anaphylactic reaction.

Courts and legislatures frequently address the issues described above. The law is in a constant state of evolution, but it is likely that the notion of duty, breach, causation, and damages will remain the bedrock of this country's tort law. The concepts are easy to understand but difficult to apply in the real world.

Evolution of Medical Malpractice

While it is possible to trace a case asserting medical negligence back to 1374 in England and to 1794 in the United States, such cases were relatively rare prior to the 1960s. There were several reasons for this:

- Society's view of a physician, prior to the 1960s, was that of a trusted member of the family who, through years of service to the family, built up such confidence and goodwill that it would be virtually unthinkable to sue him. This was an era in which a family received most of its care from one doctor. Doctors were generally held in high esteem, and juries were inclined to find in favor of physicians. That was before the explosion of specialized practices.

- In earlier times, if a patient did sue, the plaintiff would encounter the "locality rule," which required that another physician be willing to testify regarding the "standard of care" in that locality. The courts, at that time, held that a physician could criticize and testify against another physician *only* if familiar with the customs and practices of medicine in that particular locale. The rationale for the locality rule was first expressed in the case of *Small v. Howard* (1880), 128 Mass. 131, in the following language: "It is a matter of common knowledge that a physician in a small country village does not usually make a specialty of surgery, and however well informed he may be in the theory of all parts of his profession, he would, generally speaking, be but seldom called upon as a surgeon to perform difficult operations. He would have but few opportunities of observation and practice in that line such as public hospitals or large cities would afford. The defendant was applied to, being the practitioner in a small village, and we think it was correct to rule that 'he was bound to possess that skill only which physicians and surgeons of ordinary ability and skill, practicing in similar localities, with opportunities for no larger experience, ordinarily possess; and he was not bound to possess that high degree of art and skill possessed by eminent surgeons practicing in large cities, and making a specialty of the practice of surgery."

  As a practical matter, this would have required that a plaintiff's expert witness be a physician from the same locale in order to testify against the other. The "locality rule" represented a real and powerful roadblock to asserting claims of medical negligence.

- Consequent to the locality rule, another roadblock to plaintiffs arose, the so-called "conspiracy of silence" among doctors. Since the locality rule required a patient to prove that local standards of medical care had been breached, physicians simply would not testify against their peers and colleagues in any given locality. Thus, a patient plaintiff would be unable to secure the requisite expert testimony related to the local standards of care and could not prevail in a suit.

During the American cultural revolution of the 1960s, many of society's time-honored ways of thinking and acting underwent radical change. Populations were more mobile and people were no longer willing to blindly accept the declarations of their government, big business, and other societal institutions. The relationship between physician and patient was no exception. Changes occurred both inside and outside the physician/patient relationship that would drastically alter the way in which each party viewed the other.

The way in which people received medical services began to change. The era of specialization meant that people were no longer receiving all of their medical services from "the family doctor." There were now the cardiologist, the nephrologist, the neurologist, the orthopedist, etc. Absent long-standing personal relationships, people were more likely to question their doctors and to consult lawyers about possible legal recourse.

Societal skepticism toward unfamiliar doctors encouraged the erosion and ultimate elimination of the locality rule. It was the courts that had created the locality evidentiary rule, so it was up to the courts to decide if the rule still fit the real-world practice of medicine. In Ohio, for example, the rule was overturned by the Ohio Supreme Court in the case of *Bruni v. Tatsumi* (1976), 46 Ohio St.2d 127. In that case the plaintiff presented the testimony of a board-certified neurosurgeon who practiced in Columbus, Ohio. He had been critical of the care rendered by the defendant, a board-certified neurosurgeon who practiced in Canton, Ohio, but at trial he stated he did not have an opinion "on anything that happened in Canton." At the conclusion of the case, the defendant moved the court to dismiss the case, arguing that the plaintiff had failed to provide any testimony as to the standard of care specifically applicable to Canton, Ohio. The trial court agreed with this argument and dismissed the case. The Ohio Supreme Court ultimately rejected this argument and the "locality rule" as not being consistent with then modern methods of teaching and practicing medicine.

In explaining the historical context of the "locality rule," the Court wrote: "The basis for this rule was that a physician at that time in a small town lacked the opportunity to keep abreast of the advances in the medical profession and that he did not have the most modern facilities to provide care and treatment for his patients. Under those circumstances it would be unfair to hold such a doctor to the same standards of care as doctors who have such opportunities and facilities in larger cities."

The Court went on to say: "Admittedly, there was ample justification for a local-standard rule then and for many years following. But in this modern era, means of transportation facilitate opportunities for physicians and surgeons from small communities to attend up-to-date medical seminars; the general circulation of medical journals makes new developments readily available to them and they can easily communicate with the most advanced medical centers in the country."

The Court cited with approval a previous study concerning modern methods utilized in the medical profession: "The editorial board of the *Stanford Law Review*, in 1962, conducted a survey to determine to what extent the practice of medicine, within each of the 19 then recognized specialties of the American Medical Association, is similar throughout the country. Letters and questionnaires were sent to each of the American Specialty Boards, the American Medical Association, the American Hospital Association, the publishers of medical specialty journals, and the medical specialty societies. The conclusion reached was as follows: "On the basis of the existence of standardized requirements for certification, subscriptions to medical specialty journals, medical specialty societies, and statements from American Specialty Boards, it is concluded that the practice of medicine by certified specialists within most medical specialties is similar throughout the country. 14 Stanford L.Rev. 884, 887 (1961-62)."

Based upon this information, the Court concluded: "So, the locality rule has been increasingly eroded as being antiquated and unrealistic, especially in the medical specialties field.... Accordingly, the standard of care in this case is that owed to a patient by the community of neurosurgeons. Geographical conditions or circumstances do not control either the standard of the specialist's care or the competence of the expert's testimony".

Ohio was not alone in rejecting the locality rule. Similar decisions in other states resulted in patients' having access to physicians from all around the country to serve as expert witnesses in malpractice cases against physicians. A cardiologist from Illinois could testify that the actions of a cardiologist in Michigan deviated from accepted standards of care, even if the Illinois physician was not licensed by the state of Michigan. The requirement that the patient's expert be familiar with the requisite "standard of care" remains, but the standard is national, not local.

Increased access to expert witnesses resulted in more cases being filed against physicians. The allure of potentially large verdicts drew the interest of attorneys, who recognized that, although medical malpractice cases were still difficult, the potential returns often justified the investment of time, money, and resources. Large verdicts were often sensationalized in the media and served to provide the attorneys with an ever-growing number of clients who were dissatisfied with their medical providers.

By the late 1970's, the explosion of malpractice cases was of grave concern to physicians and to the insurance companies that indemnified them. An increase in the number and the size of verdicts and awards caused insurance premiums to skyrocket. Some insurance companies stopped writing malpractice insurance, while many others threatened to do so unless drastic tort reform changes were enacted. Without adequate insurance protection, many physicians stated that they were simply not going to expose their personal assets and were simply not going to practice medicine. State legislatures recognized this as an untenable situation, and many began passing "tort reform" legislation designed to curb the number of cases being filed and placing caps on the amount of monetary damages recoverable in malpractice cases.

A "medical malpractice crisis" remains a major concern to physicians, their insurers, legislators, and many other groups. It is the quintessential political debate with passionate proponents on both sides, one claiming that without additional reforms the very fabric of our medical system is threatened with extinction while the other side claims that all reforms do is deny injured people their just right to compensation just so insurance companies can enjoy greater profits. The debate will likely continue into the foreseeable future. Where it will end is anyone's guess.

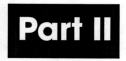

Implementing Specific Preventive Strategies

Preventing Malpractice Claims: The Science and the Art

Prevention of medical malpractice suits requires physicians to clearly understand the scope of their practices, their duties to patients, the responsibilities that they bear for the acts of their employees or subordinates, and their personal relationships with their patients. With a broad knowledge of these elements, doctors can reduce their legal exposures dramatically. Doing a comprehensive analysis of practice procedures can lower your risks substantially. We will address several practice pitfalls below that can easily be avoided at very little cost and effort. Remember Benjamin Franklin's "An ounce of prevention is worth a pound of cure."

Abnormal Laboratory Reports

Have you ever discovered a report in the record of which you knew nothing but that had a significant effect on the management of a patient? It's very disturbing when lack of awareness has led to a delay in the management of the patient's illness with adverse health effects. The fact is that this occurs more often than it should because many medical practices have no standard procedure for processing laboratory results. There is a need for prioritizing in the realm of medical reports. Both normal and abnormal results should be perused by the attending physician and then initialed and dated before being filed in the chart. Abnormal results need to be flagged and not filed permanently until the attending physician has acted upon the information.

We suggest that a copy file or logbook be established in your office and that it be reviewed weekly to follow what is being done about abnormal results. We suggest that an individual with a medical education, such as a nurse, be made responsible for the initial report file or log, but it is *ultimately the physician's responsibility,* no matter who is assigned the job. When appropriate follow up has occurred, the copy can be removed from the file or the note can be struck from the logbook. The main thing is that appropriate follow up has commenced. Appropriate follow up includes advising the patient of the results and devising a care plan. This is all part of keeping the patient informed and participating in the care process. Failure to be aware of laboratory results is very damaging and can be easily interpreted by a court as negligence.

Relying on Other Physicians and Laboratories

A clinician has the right to rely on the accuracy of reports provided by other medical specialists unless there is clear reason to suspect that the report is inaccurate or, in some way, flawed. If, for example, a physician receives a Pap smear reported as normal on a patient whose last two cytologic interpretations were reported as revealing "moderate dysplasia," there is good reason to question the report, and thus follow up is required. "Clinical correlation recommended" is a common caveat placed on laboratory and radiology reports and is there simply as a CYAWP protection for the provider of the data. Such notations are used, theoretically, to protect them from adverse consequences of flawed data. On the whole, when a physician *acts in good faith* by relying on data provided by a qualified colleague or certified laboratory, there should be no concern about personal liability.

As a corollary to the issue of *acting in reliance or acting in good faith* on a specialist's report, the clinician needs to note that, when a consultant or laboratory specialist makes a suggestion for further testing, scheduled follow ups, or additional procedures, a new care responsibility has come into effect. The follow-up advice of a consultant places a burden on the patient's attending physician to comply with the recommendation or to demonstrate good reason for not pursuing the advice. Failure to follow up on such recommendations puts the attending physician in legal peril should the patient develop complications that could have been avoided or mitigated by pursuing the advice of the consultant. Common examples of follow-up recommendations are found on radiologic, mammographic and cytologic reports.

Duty to Disclose

If a patient's laboratory work is abnormal, the attending physician is responsible for advising the patient regarding the abnormality and its significance. That may be accomplished in several ways, but however if it is done, it must be done in a timely manner. The best way to do it is face to face, but telephone communication is acceptable if it is done with care and sensitivity. Blurting out bad news on the phone can be devastating to a patient. If it is not possible to have a personal interview to deal with the problem and the patient cannot be reached by phone, a letter to the last known address is required to fulfill the physician's legal responsibility to the patient. Some people suggest sending a certified letter, but that is not the basic requirement of most jurisdictions. The letter may be sent through regular mail channels but we suggest that if that is done, a U.S. Postal Service Certificate of Mailing be purchased to provide proof of your effort to contact the patient. It is essential to keep a copy of the letter in the chart, and remember to make commemorative chart notations when personal interviews or phone conversations occur.

How to Avoid Staff-Created Malpractice Problems

Ancillary Staff

It is important for everyone in a physician's practice to understand clearly just who is authorized to practice medicine and give medical advice in the group. Receptionists, transcriptionists, bookkeepers, aids, and medical assistants are *not* licensed to practice medicine. It is up to the physicians within a practice to identify which of the personnel are authorized to provide direct medical services and give medical advice or instructions. The bottom line is that any medical advice or other practice-related acts that are performed under the umbrella of a medical practice are the responsibility of the physician(s). Anything that might be considered negligent is placed at the door of the doctor(s) in charge. For that reason, it is extremely important that ancillary staff be specifically educated regarding the nature of their jobs, their scope of responsibilities, and the limits on their interactions with patients. There have been cases in which doctors have been sued because a staff member dispensed treatment advice over the phone to a very sick patient. It is best practice to have all calls related to the care and treatment of patients referred directly to a physician or other medically qualified staff member, such as a designated R.N., for triage, medical advice, and care decisions.

Ancillary medical practice personnel are employed to support physicians in the medically related activities of a practice. Their jobs should be structured to facilitate contact between doctor and the patient, not to shield the doctor from contact, protect the doctor's time, or to give medical advice. Practice staff should be responsible for conveying information from patients to physicians or other designated staff with medical education and relay information back to patients. The conveyance of information back to patients is entirely appropriate, but care must be taken in the accuracy of the communications. It is good practice for all interactions between patients and doctors to be placed in the chart. A written and dated note, added to the chart, should reflect the patient's complaints, the discussion with the doctor (i.e., condition discussed, orders noted), and the information related to the patient.

Care Protocols

Many large practices are deluged, e.g., during the flu season, with calls that they cannot possibly answer individually. What can they do to fulfill their responsibilities of care to those patients? We suggest that they establish patient care protocols (triage) for certain types of complaints that can be managed by specially trained nurses or physician assistants. When calls come in with complaints that fit the protocol guidelines, the nurse or assistant can give the appropriate care instructions. The caveat that, if symptoms worsen, the patient must be seen by a physician as soon as possible must be emphasized. Any calls that do not meet the triage protocol guidelines must be presented to the doctor for early assessment. Calls that do meet the guidelines should be reviewed by the physician as soon as possible, dated and initialed. The notes should include the name of the patient, the caller's name, all appropriate history, advice given, and telephone numbers or other ways of reaching the calling party or patient. The physician must take an active role in ensuring the quality of the care rendered to his or her patients and cannot delegate the care to non-physicians without inviting significant legal consequences.

Ancillary Personnel Job Descriptions

Physicians should provide detailed job descriptions for each position in a practice. Each job description should detail job responsibilities, physical requirements, necessary credentials, work hours, benefits, salary, etc. It should clearly indicate the types of information that may be passed on to patients and what procedures are to be followed in the case of urgent or emergency situations. This advice pertains to both face-to-face and telephone contacts with patients. Working in a medical office does not imbue a non-medical employee with the knowledge to render medical advice.

Professional Staff

Nurses and other qualified staff members may participate in eliciting histories in a practice and may give advice commensurate with their training and experience, but even that should be specified. Nurse practitioners and physician's assistants have greater latitude in what they may do, but when associated with a medical practice, their specific duties and practice parameters should be clearly outlined.

The dangers of gratuitous medical advice must be kept fresh in the minds of the lay staff; the dangers should be raised at regular intervals, because staff members do forget and frequently unrealistic demands are placed upon them by patients. It is up to the responsible physician to regularly survey his or her staff and the jobs that they perform to ensure that he or she is not being placed in harm's way by well-meant but legally dangerous practices in the office.

Scheduling Physician Time

Scheduling appointments creates contractual obligations on a physician and the practice. In essence, a physician or practice agrees, through the receptionist who acts as the agent in scheduling, to provide the patient adequate time and opportunity to consider a reasonable number of medical questions or concerns at a given visit. Patients expect to have adequate time with a physician to deal with the concerns that they have. It is important for physicians to analyze the adequacy of office time to produce reasonable scheduling patterns in conjunction with the practice receptionist. Each time an appointment is made, a contract has actually been made on behalf of the physician for the care of a specific patient. In this time of advanced diagnostic technologies, it is important that a patient not be deprived of the chance for an early diagnosis that may have a great impact on prognosis. That opportunity to provide the needed care can be reduced when a physician, working with an overcrowded schedule, is unable to direct the amount of attention necessary to conduct a thorough patient assessment. In such cases good medical practice can be augmented by the use of trained nurses and physician's assistants to do portions of the patient work up. Patients pay for the best judgment and experience of a physician, so we advise that, when possible, it is the physician that carries out patient assessment. It's good in terms of the relationship with the patient and lowers the risk of diagnostic and treatment errors.

No matter the type of practice, scheduling is a very important issue that can make clinical practice a joy or an overwhelming burden. Just as in the case of telephone procedures, the physician(s) in charge should set policy and should specify exactly how scheduled appointments should be handled. One thing that should be made clear in scheduling policy is that, if there is not enough time in the physicians' schedule to see a patient with a problem within a reasonable time, the patient *must* be provided with immediate care options. If there is any doubt as to the well-being of the patient, the physician must be involved, immediately, in the scheduling or referral option.

There is no substitute for clear communication with staff regarding telephone policy and scheduling. Responsibility for the effectiveness of both activities lies squarely on the shoulders of the physician(s). Errors of both omission and commission can come back to haunt the physician should harm occur to a patient because of poorly considered policy or procedures related to patient communications.

Obligations and Burdens of Providing Preventive Care

Although physicians may not be able to perform every type of preventive care procedure in their office practices, it is their responsibility to be sure that each patient under care is made aware of appropriate screenings and preventive therapies so that they may have reasonable protection from preventable or modifiable illnesses. Thorough medical histories and physical examinations, plus appropriate laboratory tests, serve as good documentation of prudent care by physicians. Failure to appropriately document the assessments of well patients with suspicious personal or family histories is considered by some courts as being as much a breach of the physician's professional responsibility to his patient as any error of commission or omission on an ill patient.

Pap smears, mammography, lipid profiles, occult blood tests, and flexible sigmoidoscopies have become widely recognized by the general public as early interventional screening methods. An increasing proportion of the population sees as important immunizations for the prevention of communicable diseases. It behooves every physician to be aware that routinely offering patients screening procedures and immunizations appropriate to their practices is a prudent practice.

Among the causes of action most frequently brought against physicians in recent years is the failure to diagnose a variety of malignancies. The majority of the legal actions are predicated on the fact that the technology to diagnose these diseases is readily available to clinicians and that they should be utilized for the benefit of patients. Failure to offer an evaluation to an individual in an identified high-risk group for a preventable or modifiable disease has been found to be medical negligence in a number of cases. For example, failure to offer prenatal genetic screenings and counseling to high-risk couples planning pregnancies has raised issues of negligence in some jurisdictions, just as the failure to offer indicated screening tests to at-risk patients has led physicians into legal difficulties.

Legal liability can be minimized by making sure that each office has a list of practice-specific screening procedures to be offered to patients. Immunization and well-recognized health screening procedures should definitely be on the list. Patients should be offered evaluations at appropriate intervals, and, when the evaluations are performed, they should be clearly documented and the results noted. If an evaluation is refused, that should also be clearly stated in the chart. If nothing is written, courts generally assume that no offer was made, even though an oral offer may have been made and refused. If screening results are suspicious, the patient must be contacted directly, by telephone or by mail. Make note in the chart if a call is made and include a copy of the letter if communication is by mail.

As diagnostic techniques get better, the list of indicated screening procedures will continue to grow. Physicians must keep abreast of developments in areas of special risk to their patients. Consultations and referrals to appropriate colleagues when a physician is unable to perform needed tests or procedures are encouraged. Do not delay in pursuing what you feel should be done today on behalf of a patient. If you consider a test and do not pursue it, note your reason for not doing it. That will demonstrate reasonable and prudent behavior if it turns out that a "good faith" error was made.

As medical science has advanced, preventive care practices have expanded greatly. Immunizations have become so numerous that it frequently boggles the mind to recall just how to schedule them. Prophylactic treatments for certain types of problems, such as antibiotic therapy for heart valve disease and antimalarials for travelers to lands where that disease is prevalent, have become frequent challenges. Management of hypertension and lipid disorders requires familiarity with a large number of treatment options. Pap smears, newborn screenings, and cancer surveillance all require that physicians establish practice policies and procedures for well care and disease prevention. And so it goes, with more and more preventive options being available to patients through the efforts of medical science. Society and the courts view preventive care as a part of the "due diligence and prudent care" that physicians are required to provide to patients.

Dealing with Conflict

There is a common belief among physicians and their patients that the vast majority of medical malpractice claims are based on technical failures, diagnostic or therapeutic, that have caused injury to a patient. The perception that errors of omission or commission in diagnosis or treatment are the principal cause is not borne out by plaintiffs in a large percentage of cases. What does appear to be the most common cause of estrangement between patients and caregivers is a breakdown in the sense of cordiality and communication between the patient, the doctor and/or the physician's staff. Patients who bring claims against their doctors frequently complain of being disrespected, ignored, and taken for granted, or treated in a demeaning fashion. They speak of the arrogance of physicians and their staffs. Most of us know that there is nothing that makes a person angrier than being ignored, feeling victimized and defenseless. Many claims are filed to put the physician and others in health care on notice that the patient/plaintiff is neither insignificant nor powerless in the health care interaction.

The Essential Feature Is Communication

Communication is essential to good relationships. The communication between doctor and patient needs to be balanced and respectful. Physicians are placed in a position of high trust and respect by members of our society. In the past, and even in the present time, physicians have been placed on a societal pedestal and given many of the prerogatives of a parent in their dealings with patients. For centuries, doctors have called the shots in diagnosis and treatment, but, as the lay population has become more educated and sophisticated, the need for a more balanced dialog has come into play. Unfortunately, not all physicians have become aware of or are sensitive to that need and have thus suffered the devastating effects of patient-initiated legal recourse.

Respect for Patients' Autonomy

Respect between physician and patient is based on one of the most sacred principles of our society. It stipulates that every *competent adult,* with very few exceptions, has the right to personal autonomy. Every individual has the right of consent or denial of any assessment or procedure performed on his person. The procedures may be diagnostic, therapeutic, or rehabilitative. Even if the procedures are life-saving, the competent individual has the legal right of consent or denial. But, in order to consent to or decline care, the patient must be adequately informed to be able to make *prudent* and *reasonable* decisions. This is the point at which many misunderstandings and disagreements between doctors and patients begin. Doctors are busy and the time demands of some patients can seem unreasonable, but the physician must understand that poor communication is an almost certain road to conflict and a possible professional disaster.

Every physician needs to think his way through the requirements of what constitutes equitable interaction with patients. One must decide what is required in order to provide the patient with a satisfactory understanding of what he is facing in terms of his medical care. The physician, after establishing the doctor-patient relationship, assumes the duty to use reasonable skill and knowledge in determining what ails the patient and then has the duty to pursue a prudent plan of management. In these processes, the patient needs to be included in the decision making by being told the nature of the diagnostic and/or therapeutic process—its risks, benefits, and alternatives. The patient needs to know these things to be able to reasonably cooperate in the process. The docile, uninformed, and blindly compliant patient does not do himself or his physician a service. The full weight of diagnostic/therapeutic success or failure in that case rests entirely on the physician. Should results be poor, a docile patient can become a tiger as a plaintiff. Establishing a care partnership with the patient is a reasonable and prudent plan for every health care provider.

Dealing with the Family and Friends

The patient is frequently not the only person in the care relationship with whom the physician has to communicate. In dealing with minors, there are parents and with the elderly, there are children. There are also issues of spouses, siblings, and significant others. How does one deal with all of these people? The three word answer is *"patiently and respectfully."* While recognizing the need to observe the right of the patient to personal privacy, physicians should be helpful, courteous, and patient with those who care about the patient as well. In some circumstances, that starts with advising them of the limits of the physician's ability to disclose detail of the patient's care. Some states allow spouses to be informed of a patient's condition without specific waiver of the right of confidentiality, but others hold the right to privacy sacrosanct unless waived specifically. The patient's right of privacy needs to be respected unless specifically waived. This issue of privacy seems to arise most often in the management of adolescents with sexually related problems. Parents often resent the state statute-based independence of their children in such matters.

If a patient does give the physician the right to disclose details of his condition to others, the physician faced with many concerned friends and relatives may wish to request that the family and friends choose a spokesperson with whom he can speak candidly and allow that spokesperson to convey the information necessary to the others involved. However it is done, personal contact demonstrates caring, concern, and professionalism to the patient and his or her loved ones.

Dealing with Anger and Frustration

Anger and frustration are fairly common manifestations of patients and their families during an illness. It is wise for the physician to understand that anger and frustration expressed at times of stress are the result of fear and a sense of powerlessness. When those anxieties are not managed well, they can escalate into unnecessary conflict and ultimately into legal ugliness. The prudent physician should make every effort to speak with the patient and family often and in understandable terms. Medical jargon can be an alienating factor to a fearful patient and/or family. The physician should be forthright, even when the condition of the patient is in question. Many a good physician has been sued because he or she failed to "be honest or to show concern and compassion" to the family during an illness of a loved one. A few well-chosen words, a pat on the shoulder, and regular visitations provide patients and their families with a sense of comfort because they have visible evidence that the doctor cares.

When anger is manifested, it is a good idea for the physician to confront it directly. It is not a good idea to ignore it or to avoid it. The patient and/or family needs to deal with it, and so does the physician who plans to continue to contribute to the care of the patient. The best way to deal with it is to acknowledge that it is present. The physician should ask those concerned what it is that is creating the anger and try to understand what can be done to deal with it. Sometimes, the anger is not directed against the physician at all, but, if it is not confronted, that will not be known. If there are things that the physician can do to allay the anger, the family should be told what it is that will be done to deal with the objectionable situations. If the anger is directed toward the physician, it must be determined if the doctor can correct the problem. If the physician cannot allay the problem, he should inform the patient and family of appropriate care options and allow them to obtain alternative care. This must be done in a non-hostile, professional manner.

The hardest thing about physicians and anger situations is that doctors often fail to consider the breadth of the causes of the anger and they take it personally. There is a need to view the hostility in a stressful health care situation as an understandable clinical manifestation of perceived victimization and powerlessness on the part of patient and/or family. If a doctor can successfully deal with these types of situations and maintain a high quality of professionalism, he is truly a competent, self-assured professional. The most important point is that the physician must not become a party to the hostility. Despite the pressures, he must be controlled, polite, respectful, and, again, professional. He must not try to hide or to avoid the issues or the hostile party or parties in the situation. Avoidance is frequently interpreted as neglect or arrogance.

There are times when anger is manifested through uncooperative or disruptive behavior. When a patient behaves in that way, it is frequently due to a need to deny illness. Again, confrontation of the behavior, along with an explanation of the risks involved and how the patient may rectify the situation is important. In these types of situations, careful chart documentation is of great risk management benefit to the physician.

Advance Directives

Advance directives for health are legally binding documents prepared for an individual by an attorney in anticipation of a possible future health care-related event. Many states make state-authorized forms available to citizens wishing to express their wishes regarding health care. The *Durable Power of Attorney for Health* and the *Living Will* have been established to give persons a say in their own health care should they be unable to express their desires at the time when grave decisions regarding health care must be made.

Durable Power of Attorney and Medical Care

Most states over the past decade have instituted durable power of attorney legislation. A durable power of attorney is an *advance directive* that allows a competent individual to appoint another person (not necessarily a lawyer; it may be a friend or family member) to act as his/her *Attorney in Fact for Health Care*. The Attorney in Fact is committed to act in the best interests of the patient and carry out his or her wishes regarding health care decisions. The Durable Power of Attorney has some limitations on the breadth of discretion of the appointed attorney, but it is an excellent vehicle for a person to express his or her wishes regarding health care should he or she become unable to express them. Its duration varies, depending on state statutes, and it is easily revoked if the patient implementing it has a change of mind. It is an excellent document for citizens who wish to have trusted friends or family maintain control over their destiny should they become disabled and unable to speak for themselves. The Durable Power of Attorney for Health is an effective way to deal with unforeseen catastrophic eventualities in one's life. If a person wishes that everything medically possible be done for him or her in case of severe illness or accident, it can be clearly stated. If limits on care are desired, that too can be indicated.

In 1990, the U.S. Supreme Court decision in the Nancy Cruzan case *(Cruzan v. Director, Missouri Department of Health)* raised a number of important questions for citizens concerned with their health care should they become unable to personally state their care preferences. It was decided by the U.S. Supreme Court that mentally competent individuals do have a right to limit, refuse, or discontinue care and in effect accept death as an alternative to medical care. The Court also ruled that each state has the authority to determine the boundaries within which such decisions can be made. In essence the Cruzan case was treated by the Court as a state's rights case.

In that case Nancy Cruzan had been unconscious and in a vegetative state for several years; the Court supported the position of the Supreme Court of the State of Missouri. That Court had ruled that, in the absence of the written wishes of the patient to discontinue life support-systems and nutrition in the case of total disability, the family of the patient has no inherent right to discontinue those systems. The Supreme Court of the State of Missouri had ruled previously that the family's judgment could not be substituted for Nancy's and that passing or casual comments made by her when she was well and able were not sufficient to clearly establish her wishes.

In the past, a number of states have allowed substitute judgments based on the clearly stated preferences of incapacitated patients prior to their disabilities. Family members, friends, or court-appointed guardians have been allowed to act as surrogates in the best interests of patients. Several legal tests have been used by courts to protect the interests of patients. Among those tests is the "prudent and reasonable person test," which assesses what others in similar circumstances would do. There is also a legal test to establish, by the personal knowledge of acquaintances, the wishes of the patient. In the *Cruzan* case, these and similar tests were set aside, and the state's preeminence to determine the guidelines within which such decisions can be made was asserted. It is interesting that, once the state's right issue was resolved, the Cruzan family was allowed to remove Nancy's feeding tube, after which she died relatively soon.

States have, in many areas, the authority to determine that some public interests override personal interests. States' interests supersede individual interests in many areas of commerce, property, and taxation. The *Cruzan* case added a new perspective to the level of authority that a state can exert over a family in decision making regarding irreversibly impaired family members. In a mitigating gesture, the U.S. Supreme Court allowed that the clearly stated desires of the patient in regard to life support and sustenance, in a written form such as a living will, would be sufficient to establish and allow the wishes of that person to be carried out.

The Living Will

A living will is another advance directive that provides the individual concerned with his or her health care additional force of law. The living will is a directive, produced by a competent individual (the testator), that indicates directly to the physician how he or she wants his or her medical care managed if he or she becomes terminally ill and unable to express his or her will. The intent of the living will is to provide patients with personal autonomy as it relates to health care. This document supersedes the authority of the durable power of attorney if or when the patient's condition becomes terminal or if there is a high probability of becoming "permanently vegetative." The testator may indicate the types of care that may be employed and whether he or she will agree to any therapy, considered extraordinary or not. The courts have defined extraordinary care generally as modalities that go beyond what is normally considered comfort care. A number of courts have ruled IVs, airways, and nasogastric feedings as extraordinary care and subject to the patient's competent refusal.

Living Will legislation requires that there be a competent testator and a witness or witnesses who have *no interest* in the estate of the testator. Family members, beneficiaries, the patient's physician, and other caretakers may not be witnesses. Competent patients and even some incompetent patients have been granted autonomy by the courts when it has been clear that they appreciated the consequences of their actions and the requested acts are in concert with the patients' established behaviors and preferences.

Physicians should be aware of the living will status of their patients. A copy of a Durable Power of Attorney and a Living Will in the patient's chart is a good practice. If a physician is not willing to participate in the choices of a patient, he or she is not required to act in a way adverse to his or her own beliefs, but should notify the patient and the family of his or her position and be willing to withdraw from care if necessary.

Living Wills have grown in importance to patients who wish to have personal autonomy in individual care since the Nancy Cruzan case. That case emphasized the need for a patient who is terminally ill or in a vegetative state to have a clearly expressed opinion, preferably in writing, relating to terminal care prior to that state being reached. Some states require the "expressed statement" to be in writing in "statutorily prescribed language."

Although there have not been a large number of medical claims concerning Advance Directives, there have been enough to warrant comment on the potential legal consequences of disregarding the provisions of a Durable Power of Attorney, a Living Will, or do not resuscitate (DNR) orders.

Any health care provider who disregards the clearly expressed desire concerning what medical measures a patient is willing to undergo potentially faces a claim of medical battery. The consequences for the battery would include any damages arising from the battery inflicted on the patient. Likewise, the provider may face licensing sanctions and/or suspension or revocation of hospital privileges.

Despite the legal standing of Advance Directives, the course that the courts will follow is not fully clear. A pair of examples in the Ohio law will demonstrate the point.

What are the "damages" when a provider disregards a patient's desire not to be resuscitated or the terms of a living will stating he does not want any life-sustaining treatment in the face of a terminal condition? In *Anderson v. St. Francis/St. George Hospital*, an 82-year-old cardiac patient was admitted to the hospital. He told his personal physician that he did not want to be resuscitated, as his wife had seriously deteriorated following resuscitation. The doctor entered a "NO CODE BLUE" on the order sheet, yet kept the patient on a cardiac monitor. Three days after the admission, the patient suffered ventricular tachycardia. A nurse defibrillated him and succeeded in reviving him. She did so, in part, on the basis of the fact that the patient was on a monitor. Two days later, the patient suffered a paralyzing stroke, requiring extensive care until his death two years later.

A lawsuit sought damages for the hospital's failure to obey the "NO CODE BLUE" order. The Ohio Supreme Court recognized that the negligent disregard of such an order may justify nominal damages or any damages actually caused by the life-sustaining treatment. However, the court rejected the contention that the hospital was liable for prolonging the patient's life, including the suffering of the subsequent stroke. The court held that defining the harm giving rise to damages was the stumbling block in recognizing a claim for "wrongful living." It would require a jury to decide the relative merits of "being versus non-being," or, as another court stated, "life, however impaired and regardless of any attendant expenses, cannot rationally be said to be a detriment when compared to the alternative of non-existence."

In a similar case, *Allore v. Flowers Hospital*, a claim was made against a cardiologist and a nurse, asserting that they had disregarded the patient's living will on file with the hospital, which directed that no life-sustaining treatment be administered if he was in a terminal condition. The cardiologist and the nurse were unaware of the living will and proceeded to intubate and then ventilate the patient when he was diagnosed with pulmonary edema. The patient lived another two days. The court rejected the claim for wrongfully prolonging the patient's life, citing the *Anderson* case. The court would have permitted recovery for damages that were actually related to the alleged battery itself (intubation/ventilation) or nominal damages. However, the plaintiff sought only damages for the patient's pain, suffering, mental anguish and unnecessary medical expenses, all of which were incurred because of prolongation of the patient's life.

To avoid being involved in similar claims, health care providers should certainly become aware of whether such advance directives exist and then seek to comply with the patient's desires. Hospital admission forms typically inquire as to the existence of living wills and/or durable powers of attorney, and such notations should not be disregarded. Moreover, a thorough and compassionate discussion with family members is also recommended as a means of reducing the stress and anguish that always accompany such decisions.

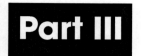
Part III

Physician Responsibilities

Informed Consent

What Is It?

Informed consent is an important element in many medical malpractice cases. By law the competent patient has absolute control over his or her body and so has the right to make a fully informed decision about any procedure to be undertaken on his or her person. A patient does not need to have every conceivable risk disclosed but should be made aware of the nature of the procedure, its risks and benefits as well as reasonable alternatives to the suggested procedure. Most important, the patient must be made aware of any significant procedural risk to life or limb. These are called material risks. Before this potential claim is discussed, it is important to understand its legal elements.

A claim based on a lack of informed consent has three elements that must be established by a patient/plaintiff at trial:

- The physician failed to disclose or discuss with the patient the material risks and inherent dangers related to the procedure.

- The undisclosed risks or dangers that should have been disclosed occurred and are the proximate cause of injury to the patient.

- A reasonable person in the patient's position "would have decided against the procedure or would have selected an alternative procedure" if the material risks and dangers had been disclosed.

The law regarding informed consent is not uniform across the country. Each state jurisdiction has developed its own policy regarding what is required in order to be in conformity with its informed consent standards. Despite a lack of uniformity in the specifics of the rules and laws dealing with consent, the legal premises on which the courts act are very similar. The paragraphs below provide a reasonable set of guidelines for physicians to follow.

The Reasonable Man Standard

The "reasonable man" standard is applicable to this claim. It is up to the jury to determine what a reasonable man would do. It is not sufficient for the patient simply to state that he or she would not have elected to have the procedure if the risks had been explained. If each of the three elements is proven, the plaintiff's claim will be heard before the jury. It is important to note that it is the plaintiff's burden to prove all three claims. If any of the three elements is not proven, the claim fails. Because of the heavy burden of proof that is placed on the plaintiff, suits based solely on informed consent are rare, but it is a potential claim in every malpractice case. Reasonable care taken by a physician to inform a patient of pertinent risks, benefits, and alternatives will, in general, prevent this claim.

Office Informed Consent

Informed consent is not necessary for routine office calls or examinations, but, if any invasive procedures are to be done, it is wise to get consent. We recommend that physicians obtain informed consent (IC) from the patient for any procedure performed in office that poses a risk of harm to the patient. Although we suggest that a consent form be signed, consent can be oral if the patient is competent. If it is oral, a note should be placed on the chart that the patient was informed of the nature of the procedure and advised of risks, benefits, and alternatives. A reasonable way of dealing with a verbal consent is to write or type your statement on the chart and have the patient sign it along with you. When dealing with a minor or an incompetent, written consent from a parent or a custodian is strongly recommended. An attorney can draft a simple consent form for your office to use when minors or legally incompetent patients are to have procedures performed at the time of an office visit.

Hospital Informed Consent

The hospital medical record needs to reflect that risks, benefits, and alternatives to a procedure have been explained to and have been understood by the patient. If there is no regular written consent on the record, a notation, by the physician, in the care notes is generally sufficient to overcome a claim of lack of informed consent and enables him or her to testify at trial about his or her habit and custom in discussing this matter with patients. It is not wise to rely on a hospital's general consent form when caring for a hospitalized patient. We strongly suggest that physicians performing procedures in hospital obtain the consent themselves, but there are exceptions. In some settings, the consent may be obtained by a nurse or an assistant. It is important that the physician be certain that the person obtaining the consent has adequate training and experience in obtaining consents and can provide adequate information to the patient or his or her representative regarding the procedure to be performed, its risks, benefits, and alternatives. When the physician's procedural note is written, it should be noted that risks, benefits, and alternatives of the procedure were explained to the patient prior to the procedure and that these elements were understood, with the patient agreeing to proceed. If the record is silent on this issue, you are subject to the argument that "if it isn't written, it probably didn't occur." The best practice is to note the discussion in the chart.

We have, over the years, seen physicians who present standard informed consent forms to the patient that include extensive lists of possible risks of a procedure. This is not an unreasonable practice, but it is subject to the risk that an unlisted complication may arise. If a prepared list of any type is to be used, be certain that the most likely and life-threatening risks (the material risks) are highlighted and clearly discussed. Leave yourself wiggle room with a qualifying statement in the IC, such as, "There may be other unspecified risks, but I agree to proceed with a clear and true understanding of the major risks explained to me which I accept." In general, the more complicated and risky a procedure, the more the notes should reflect the risk/benefit/alternatives discussion.

The General Rules of Informed Consent

The general rules that need to be followed are:

- The extent of disclosure to the patient depends on several factors and is inversely proportional to the necessity of the procedure. The greater the immediate risk to life and limb, the lower the requirement for extensive detail. In the case of an elective procedure, a detailed explanation of all of the material aspects of the procedure should be provided. In the case of a procedure or treatment where "life or limb" may be at risk, enumeration of major risks may be all that is required. In critical emergencies, very little or no consent may be required, particularly if the patient is unconscious. In the case of minors or incompetents at immediate risk of "life or limb," no consent is required if a parent or another responsible person is not available to provide it. Under conditions of extremes, if a patient denies consent for "life or limb" saving treatment, a court with appropriate jurisdiction may grant consent for medical care despite refusal by the patient, depending on how the court views the patient's and the state's interests in the matter.

- It is the responsibility of the physician prescribing the treatment or carrying out the procedure for which the patient is giving consent to acquire the consent and provide appropriate disclosures. If the responsibility is delegated to another, the attending physician may become liable for any failures of the appointed surrogate (vicarious liability) should there be any.

Battery is a cause of action that may be raised if no consent is acquired. If consent is acquired for a specifically identified procedure or treatment and another procedure or treatment is performed, battery remains a cause of action. In those cases, such as an operation on the wrong hip, no consent was obtained for the procedure, and thus it entails an "unauthorized touching," which is, by tort law definition, a battery. Under the circumstance in which the appropriate procedure is being carried out and an emergency, requiring additional effort, arises, a physician has the responsibility to extend his procedure or therapy to the benefit of the patient without specific consent.

In summary, the patient should be given a fair explanation of risks and benefits of the proposed treatment or procedure, reasonable alternatives should be mentioned, questions should be answered, the patient should be advised of his option to withdraw, and the facts should be documented. The patient's signature helps to validate the process.

Vicarious Liability

General Concept

Vicarious liability sounds like a charge that might be brought against a community peeping Tom, but it is really a term used to describe the imputation of neglect to another person not directly involved in an allegedly negligent act. We are all aware that corporations are not people, although they are run by people. If a company employee or agent injures another, the employee and/or the agent are responsible, as is the company, provided that the employee/agent was operating within the scope of his employment. The purpose of this imputation of fault is to ensure that an injured party has the right to a full recovery from the entity directing the employee's actions. We are all familiar with the concept of corporate responsibility. It is usually because the company has assets and insurance (deep pockets) while employees may not.

Respondeat Superior

The common law test under which vicarious liability is determined is that "one individual or entity possesses the power of the direction and control of another's actions." Thus, if one has the right to direct and control an employee, he is responsible for the actions of that employee. The only requirement is that the employee be acting within the scope of his employment and under the control of another individual or corporate entity.

The common law has long held that one who derives the most benefit from the provision of a service to another bears the burden of responsibility for that service. Anything that an agent or employee does wrong may be ascribed to the responsible party (the boss). The legal doctrine of "respondeat superior" is based on the tenet that the *captain of the ship* is responsible for all that occurs aboard. Whatever occurs within the scope of the specified circumstances, whether under direct supervision or not, reflects on the captain of the ship. In the not-too-distant past, it did not matter whether a negligent act was committed by a person directly under the authority and pay of the person in charge or working for him in the capacity of a "loaned servant"; he still assumed responsibility. Surgeons, in the recent past, were commonly held responsible for the acts of operating room personnel, even when they had no control over them as an employer. The surgeon was considered to be captain of the ship, and anything and everything that went on in the OR was his or her responsibility. This has changed somewhat recently, with hospitals no longer being allowed to claim that their staffs are "loaned servants" of medical staff physicians (see below).

Independent Contractors

Equipment and techniques that don't work or that work incorrectly and do injury to patients may also be a source of liability to physicians, particularly if failure could be anticipated or was foreseeable. This concept also applies to doctors who work as partners. If a partner commits malpractice, every other partner is liable for his or her actions. In an incorporated practice, the corporation is responsible for the actions of each employee.

Another issue that we want to clarify is the liability of an independent contractor. Suppose that you need a new roof and you hire a roofing contractor who shows up with workmen, ladders, etc. to perform the job. Assume also that a mailman stops by to deliver the mail and is injured when a workman accidentally drops his hammer on the mailman's head. Although the roofer is employed (paid) by you, he is certainly not under your direct control when he is on the roof. He is considered to be an independent contractor, and you have no liability for his actions while he works on your roof. This same principle applies to independent medical laboratories, MRI facilities, etc. You are generally not liable for their mistakes, as they are independent of you and they control the method and manner of operation. This is also generally true when other physicians cover your practice while you take a vacation or are away for any reason.

Agency by Estoppel: The Rules Are Changing

The concept of independent medical contractors has recently been eroded in the area of hospital liability. Most hospitals today have emergency groups that contract to cover the ED during certain hours. They also have radiology groups that read and interpret films, as well as pathology groups and house physicians that cover the hospital to provide the services necessary for the hospital to represent itself as a full-service hospital.

In the past, hospitals have been able to avoid liability for malpractice by contracting for services with physicians and claiming that they were independent contractors. The contracts were often produced to substantiate their claim. In recent years, the courts have ruled that most patients go to a given hospital for treatment, either in the ED or as an inpatient, and believe that the hospital is the provider of the care rather than the care's being rendered by groups of independent contractors. The law in many areas is changing and holding hospitals liable when a patient looks to the hospital as the provider of all services rendered. This concept is called agency by estoppel.

This changing area of the law affects every physician's rights and duties if his or her practice is hospital affiliated. There is a need to discuss with counsel the special circumstances incumbent in this type of situation and the need for malpractice insurance, who will provide it and the right, if any, of the hospital to be indemnified (repaid) by you if it has to pay on your behalf because of your negligence. These and other matters might change your present contractual relationship and should be reviewed.

The relatively recent emergence of hospitalist groups that limit their patient care to hospital inpatients has created some confusion related to the concept of independent medical contractors. Hospitalists that are hospital employed are clearly the agents of the hospital. Those hospitalists that are independent practitioners and use a hospital as their work site will be, most likely, treated by the hospital as any other independent member of a medical staff. The issues regarding hospital and/or physician liabilities will focus on how a hospital represents the services provided by those independent hopitalist physicians. If the services of independent hospitalists are in any way implied to be a part of a hospitals patient care services, the issue of Agency by Estopple will certainly come into play.

Tricky Areas that Are of Concern to Group Practices

Pitting Partners against Each Other

Let's suppose that you are one of five radiologists practicing in a local hospital and that Dr. X misreads or fails to see a tumor on an x-ray and reads it as normal. A suit is subsequently filed against the doctor who misread the film and the radiology group. You are not specifically named in that suit, but your curiosity gets the best of you and you look at the film and see the mistake in Dr. X's interpretation. You tell no one what you saw, but you receive notice that you and the other members of the group are being subpoenaed to give depositions, although your name doesn't appear on any record. In some jurisdictions, a physician can be called and asked his opinion on the medical services rendered by a partner. This can be devastating when one is asked to testify and disagrees with a partner. Remember that the misinterpretation of an obvious lesion such as a fracture or a mass in the skull makes the jury "experts." They can see the problem and can point it out, even though they have no training. That makes them very unsympathetic toward the defendant. This matter of pitting partners against each other in court is relatively new but needs to be approached with the aid of attorneys with experience in the statutes of the state of one's practice.

Conveying Information in a Group Practice

Another area of concern is that of office practice in a group. Suppose that Dr. A writes his notes while Dr. B dictates his. On Monday, a patient comes in with severe abdominal pain. Dr. A writes a thorough note, using the SOAP format; prescribes appropriate medication; and discharges the patient. The patient returns two days later with worsening symptoms, but Dr. B only writes a few marginal notes and dictates the rest. The next day the patient returns feeling much worse; the staff is backed up and Dr. B has the day off. Not knowing what Dr. B thought or found, because the dictation has not yet been transcribed, Dr. A continues on the course set on Monday. Do you see the potential problems with this practice? What could they have done? (See "Dictated Charts," page 72, for more on this issue.)

As discussed elsewhere in this book, it is important in a group practice for each member to use the same measurements, shorthand notations, language, and format for each patient note. Every member of the group needs to be able to pick up a chart and to know exactly what the prior doctor was thinking and doing. This helps in the continuity of patient care and keeps group members from internal criticisms in malpractice cases.

Failure to Diagnose or Treat Appropriately

Failure to Diagnose

Most claims against physicians are based on the charge that the physician failed to properly diagnose or failed to properly treat a known condition. These claims are based on the premise that the physician, as an expert, should be able to arrive at the correct diagnosis of the condition that brought the patient in and should be able to appropriately treat the problem, given the tools available to the physician to solve the problem. Because there is a presumption that a patient will tell the truth to the doctor, the historical evidence in the possession of the physician, along with the physical examination, test results, and other positive or negative findings, should lead the average practitioner to the right conclusion.

Misdiagnosis and/or mistreatment of any identifiable condition is considered to be, by plaintiff's attorneys, malpractice and are the basis of many lawsuits. For example, if a patient goes to a doctor with a suspicious lump in her breast and a history of a mother and sister with breast cancer and the doctor makes the diagnosis of a non-cancerous condition without obtaining a biopsy, he is in trouble. Similarly, if a patient presents himself to the emergency department with complaints of shortness of breath, chest pain that radiates to the left shoulder and arm, sweating, and nausea, and a diagnosis of gastritis is made with the patient being sent home, that is trouble with a capital T.

Misdiagnosis Is a Big Problem

Misdiagnosis is a greater problem than mistreatment in malpractice cases. If a problem is correctly diagnosed, the chances are that it will be treated appropriately. A very great problem for physicians today is that the world of medicine is changing daily, and the physician is required to maintain the same skills and expertise as doctors in the finest educational centers. On the other hand, doctors are all too frequently called on the carpet by care managers for ordering "unnecessary tests." These many factors create ethical/economic dilemmas for the practitioner trying to manage problem patients. It is impossible to satisfy everyone's demands. As a general rule, if a diagnosis seems clear, go with it, but be sure to keep careful records that reflect your thought processes. If there are any concerns about the diagnosis, go with the first impression, but note in the record how you are proceeding to rule out other diagnostic probabilities. If the record reflects a clear and reasonable thought process in the attempt to arrive at the best diagnosis, you will generally be on safe ground.

The Standard of Care

An example of how the standard of care is established can be demonstrated in a *failure to diagnose* claim. The contention of the plaintiff is generally that the defendant physician breached his or her duty of care. The plaintiff tries to establish that the care fell below the minimum standard that other "prudent and reasonable" physicians would have exercised under the "same or similar" circumstances. A common scenario is that of a patient who presents himself to a physician for care and is not evaluated for his complaint or an inappropriate evaluation is performed. Another way that this cause of action may arise is when a problem that is not present is erroneously diagnosed and an injury ensues in the evaluation or treatment of the nonexistent problem.

The common law holds that the physician, "having held himself out as an expert" in the diagnosis and treatment of diseases, has the duty to utilize his skills in a "prudent and reasonable" manner in accord with the standards of his profession. If he fails in this duty and the patient is injured, there is "a cause of action" by the injured party. The standard of care in medical malpractice litigation is established through the testimony of physicians that practice in the specific medical field in question. If a suit is based on a urological problem then urologists are the expert witnesses that establish the professional standard of care. The standard is based on the hypothetical premise of what "a reasonable and prudent physician of similar education and experience would do under the same or similar circumstance". Each side, plaintiff and defense, produces medical experts that testify as to the standard of care of their specialty. These presentations by medical experts are heard by the jury and it is up to them to decide on the standard of care based on the testimony presented to them. Once the jury has settled on the standard, as they understand it, they decide whether the standard of care was breached or not by the defendant.

It is easy to see how important it is for the sides in a medicolegal trial to present good expert witnesses. Based on long experience, it has been our observation that juries have an uncanny record of coming up with the correct verdict in a majority of medical malpractice cases even when they do not fully understand why. Much of their perspicacity seems to be derived from their observation of what goes on in the court room. Jurors seem to sense the truth related to a case in point even when the facts of the case may not be entirely clear to them. With that in mind, it is extremely important that a defendant physician deport himself or herself professionally in court. A professional appearance during the trial, calmness during the trial proceedings and well thought out, credible testimony, directed to the jury, are major components in any successful defense.

Not Every Error or Omission Means Trouble

A physician is not liable for every diagnostic omission, but the law and standards of medical practice require that he pursue a clearly reasonable course in dealing with diagnostic questions. The physician is not expected, or required, to be perfect but must demonstrate at least a minimum level of competence compared to other physicians in his or her specialty, under "the same or similar" circumstances. The reasonableness of the process can best be established by careful documentation of the physician's encounters with the patient and of the results of all evaluations.

Failure to Treat Appropriately

The same basic elements hold true for the claim of failure to treat appropriately. In this situation, the charge is that the physician, despite a probable or obvious diagnosis, failed to proceed appropriately to treat the problem. If the physician fails to follow a reasonable course of therapy, fails to document the logic of his or her reasoning, or fails to identify clearly the type of problem with which he or she is dealing, he or she is subject to legal liability. A professional standard, which is the product of expert testimony, is used to establish the prudence and reasonableness of the defendant physician.

Avoid Liability by Clear Documentation

If these causes of action are to be avoided, physicians would be wise to subscribe to the following:

- Document the patient's history carefully.

- Document all pertinent physical and laboratory findings.

- Make an assessment of conclusions reached, based on all of the data available.

- Document progress and plans for further work-up and/or treatment.

In addition, it is good practice to get consultation when a difficult problem in diagnosis or treatment arises, because it helps to establish the physician's concern and prudence. If other than standard diagnostic or therapeutic procedures are to be followed, the fact that the patient was fully informed and in agreement with the course of action must be documented. Even in the case of standard procedures, it is a good idea to document having informed the patient of the process.

An important part of what is judged to be excellent health care is tied to the quality of the records produced by the physician on behalf of the patient. Carefully kept records reinforce memory, reveal the nature of the doctor-patient interaction, and attest to the judgment and competence of the physician. The importance of accurate, well-documented records at trial cannot be overstated.

The Differential Diagnosis

As noted above, the greatest risk today for litigation in medical practice is misdiagnosis. This is especially true in emergency medicine, cancer management, heart disease, and obstetrics. In any situation in which the differential diagnosis includes life-threatening or quality of life issues, the physician must pursue a plan that will allow him to identify and/or rule out high-risk problems. Failure to formulate and pursue a reasonable differential diagnosis forms the basis of many lawsuits against emergency department physicians, radiologists, and obstetricians. A common scenario will help to make this point. A not uncommon problem is that of a patient arriving at the ED with vague chest pain, slight sweating, and a bit of nausea and having a normal ECG. The patient gives a history of overeating and has a favorable response to a GI cocktail. The only diagnosis on the chart is dyspepsia, and no differential diagnosis is produced. If the patient is discharged with an antacid prescription and told to return if the symptoms worsen, the door has been opened to a huge liability problem. If the patient does well, there is no problem. If he dies within a short time, and an autopsy shows that he died of an MI, guess who is going to be sued. In this type of case, the ED doctor usually loses hands down because of his failure to consider and rule out a potentially life-threatening problem that should have been addressed in the differential diagnosis. The less demanding route of symptomatic treatment was taken, and there was a failure to seek out the pathology that was causing the symptoms.

Another common problem is the complaint of rectal bleeding, too often attributed to hemorrhoids, in a middle-aged patient. Commonly, an inadequate history is taken, and the patient is not thoroughly examined. Rectal examinations, proctoscopic exams and colonoscopy are not favorites among patients, but they must be done to rule out serious occult diseases. Patients with the potential for serious disease must be carefully worked up or followed with close observation. The more likely that a symptom might be due to a serious problem, the greater the clinician's responsibility to pursue a thorough work up. If one is to err, it should always be on the conservative side. Take no chance that a patient will develop a disabling or lethal problem. If the differential diagnosis includes any high-risk illnesses, the standard of care demands deliberate and well-thought-out action.

The differential diagnosis should reflect what "another reasonable and prudent physician under the same or similar circumstances" would have included in the assessment. Failure to consider and rule out a life-threatening and/or life-endangering problem is a breach of the physician's duty and will place him at legal jeopardy. Failure to fully consider the various probabilities listed in a differential diagnosis presents plaintiff's counsel with a slam dunk opportunity. The failure to produce a reasonable differential at all is also an open door to trouble.

Cases based on failure to pursue differential diagnoses are very hard to defend, because it is obvious that the condition that caused the demise of or injury to the patient was a part of the defendant's thought process. Under these circumstances juries tend not to accept explanations that relieve the defendant of the responsibility for pursuing a diagnostic alternative to the working diagnosis. This is an area of medical risk management that clinicians should concentrate on. Careful attention in the formulation and pursuit of the differential diagnosis can go a long way in preventing malpractice claims.

We cannot stress too much that good record keeping is the best defense against malpractice claims, particularly in the area of diagnostic effort. If records reflect that you are proceeding from a rational diagnosis and taking the appropriate measures to rule in or out the diagnoses in the differential, you will usually be in safe waters, but if you do not, you may well be swimming with the sharks.

Medical Battery

When one thinks of the legal term battery, the term assault also comes to mind. Assault and battery seem as inseparable as Laurel and Hardy. You can hardly think of one without the other. However, in tort law, assault is one thing and battery is another. In criminal cases the two may well be associated, but in medical circumstances they are rarely linked.

Assault is commonly thought of as a physical attack upon another, but in tort law it is either an attempt to do injury or a threat to do injury that causes the object of the attempt or threat to fear for his well-being and safety. The circumstances must be such that the victim is actually put in fear and not merely a situation in which gestures or threats are meaningless. So, in medical circumstances, it would be very rare that assault would be an issue. On the other hand, battery is the basis for a considerable number of actions against physicians.

Battery is generally misunderstood by the average citizen. The layman usually considers it to be a forceful and violent physical attack upon another individual. That is certainly the case in a criminal battery, but it is not the case in medical battery. Battery is defined in tort law as "any unauthorized touching". The part of state law that defines battery deals primarily with issues of personal space, privacy, and safety. One may not touch another individual without permission except under certain specified conditions in which authorization is granted.

There is a socially accepted idea in our culture that "familiarity" among individuals with special relationships permits touching under ordinary circumstances. That concept puts emphasis on the issue of "*unwanted* touching." Certain professions, those identified as "touching professions," of which medicine is the principal one, are allowed to touch individuals within the scope of performing services for patients. The issue, as far as professionals are concerned, is that "touching" is a part of the accepted standard of care when a "prudent and reasonable physician" touches patients in the course of diagnosis and/or treatment. Excessive familiarity or unnecessary vigor in an examination may become grounds for a claim of battery against a physician. A substantial number of actions against physicians have been raised when charges of sexual battery have been raised. We recommend that a chaperone be available for any examination of a patient of the opposite sex.

Quite commonly, medical battery charges are brought against physicians when procedures not consented to are performed on patients. Such circumstances include performance of the wrong procedure; performance of the correct procedure on the wrong patient; performance of the correct procedure on the right patient but on the wrong structure, e.g., right hip instead of left hip; and performance of a procedure on a competent patient without obtaining proper informed consent. All of these circumstances create the condition of unauthorized touching. To avoid these errors we suggest that, in the pre-operative period, prior to the pre-operative medication of any patient receiving sedation or general anesthetic, the patient be asked to mark the surgical site with a felt tipped pen and that the site be checked against the surgeons pre-operative notations for site verification.

Because touching is an integral part of the practice of medicine, patients seeking medical care are expected to understand that touching is a normal and expected part of medical evaluations. Physicians performing routine examinations are given the benefit of the doubt regarding the issue of battery unless there is evidence of notable deviations from professional standards. Those deviations include undue force in examination, sexual advances, and improper and/or unauthorized diagnostic or therapeutic procedures.

Several preventive measures can help avoid claims of medical battery. The patient should fully understand what the physician is proposing to do. In the case of a patient-requested physical examination, the average patient is considered to have "common knowledge" of the process and need not have every element of the process explained. In these situations the patient is deemed to have given *implied consent*.

If the proposed examination or treatment is out of the ordinary, the patient or his representative should be carefully apprised of the nature of the process. If the patient is a minor or otherwise incompetent, the physician has a responsibility to make the patient and his parent(s) aware of what he is doing and to obtain permission from a parent or guardian. If invasive procedures, of any kind, are to be performed, the patient should be made aware of their nature and utility and a written informed consent should be obtained. If an operative procedure is to be done, the physician should carefully explain the procedure, why it should be done, and on what structure it will be performed. Again, informed consent is an absolute requirement. When possible, identifying marks, as noted above, should be made on the patient prior to surgery in order to avoid the embarrassment and liability of operating on the wrong structure.

It is incumbent on the patient's personal physician, as the patient's advocate, to help protect him or her from battery. Primary care physicians should consult with specialty colleagues who perform invasive procedures on their patients to remind them of the patients' specific problem and the nature of the agreed-upon treatment.

Abandonment

When one thinks of abandonment, a common picture that comes to mind is of a person left alone without immediate means for self-care or protection. In a real sense that is the concept that the legal system applies to the doctor-patient relationship. At the time that a patient makes an appointment to see a physician for care, the doctor and the patient enter into an unwritten contract for care that will be in effect until the specific problem is resolved. Each time that a new problem arises, a new contract is made. Physicians, depending on their specialties, contract for the care of specific ailments. For instance, a cardiologist does not contract with a patient to manage a surgical problem. He is not responsible for other care-related contractual agreements. For family physicians, pediatricians, and general internists, the scope is broader but not unlimited.

At the time that a patient contract is made, each party assumes specific responsibilities. The patient is expected to be truthful, to be present for agreed-upon appointments, and to pay for care rendered. The physician is responsible for providing care within the range of professional standards and for being available to the patient as needs arise. If the physician is not personally available, there is an implicit responsibility for ensuring that equivalent care is available.

Because medicine is a "touching profession," a physician does not have to accept every patient who is presented to him. There are exceptions, under certain dire emergency situations such as in an emergency department or in a situation in which a critically ill patient presents at his office. Under emergency circumstances, the physician may transfer care to another qualified physician as soon as it is feasible and reasonable. Physicians may terminate the doctor-patient relationship at any time "without cause" as long as adequate notice is given to the patient. Adequate notice requires that the patient be informed, usually in writing, and that a reasonable amount of time be given to find a new source of care. Under normal circumstances, seven days is considered to be reasonable. If a letter is used to inform a patient of termination, it need not be certified. Most state statutes recognize that a posted letter, sent to the last known address, is adequate notice. A copy of the letter should be placed in the chart. In addition, the law recognizes that notice is given the day that the letter is posted, whether or not it is received. Good reason to get a USPS Certificate of Mailing when the letter is mailed.

The terminating physician may suggest other sources of care to a patient or actually participate in a referral with the intent of transferring care elsewhere. The *issue of intent* is very important, and the patient must be aware of the physician's desire to be relieved of his or her care.

Delays in providing emergency or urgent care may also be looked upon by courts as abandonment. Physicians are granted a "reasonable" amount of time to attend a patient, but it depends on the situation. Abandonment suits have been initiated in obstetrical cases in which physicians have not been on site at the time of births after having been given "reasonable notice." The same risk is incurred in other emergency situations.

Legally, the physician has a duty of care once the doctor-patient relationship commences. In the case of abandonment, the physician breaches the duty of care if and when he fails to make care available to a patient with whom he has contracted. If the patient is harmed because of the breach of that duty, there is a cause of action against the contracting physician. In essence, the patient has been left without the care and protection for which he contracted, and the law will make every effort to compensate the patient for his loss.

To protect himself, a physician may do several things to prevent abandonment. Patients must be educated to the physician's normal office schedule and to alternative coverage if the physician cannot be reached or is absent. That information may be made available orally by office personnel, via brochure, by telephone answering service or answering machine, by letter, or by a sign on the doctor's premises.

The practical reality is that a physician is responsible for the care of a patient for the duration of the contract into which he has entered. Each illness creates a new contract. The contract may be terminated by either the physician or the patient. If the physician is to terminate the contract, he must provide adequate notice, best in written form.

Confidentiality of Communication between Patient and Physician

In all states, communications between physicians and their patients are *privileged*, i.e., absolutely private and confidential. Without proper authorization, a physician cannot divulge the patient's words or conduct or the results of tests to anyone without the permission of the patient or a legally appointed representative. The confidentiality of communication holds in any situation in which the patient has an expectation of privacy. In law it is said that the *privilege applies*. The privilege applies to the physician's staff as well, and each employee must understand that confidentiality surrounds all office visits by patients. The privilege belongs to the patient and can only be waived by a competent patient, a parent or legal custodian of a minor, or a guardian of an incompetent.

A physician may not speak to an attorney about a patient or copy his chart without a written, signed, and dated authorization. A physician may convey information upon receipt of an authorization that is dated and signed by the patient. There is no requirement to investigate the authenticity of the authorization if it appears to be valid on its face. In the case in which an authorization is signed by a minor or an incompetent, the authorization should be rejected in a phone call or a written response stating the reasons that the authorization is rejected. When authorizations are received, make certain that the original is kept in the patient's chart. A copy is valid if the authorization stipulates specifically that a copy may be used. Although time is not specifically an issue, we suggest that a current authorization be requested if a prior authorization is older than 60 days.

A physician may be called on to give a deposition in a civil or a criminal case by the attorney for a patient. Although there is tacit agreement by the patient to the physician's giving testimony, it is recommended that the physician ask counsel to mail or bring a fresh authorization to the deposition. This may prove unnecessary, but it is good practice.

Privileged communication, a long-respected tradition in western cultures, purports to allow full disclosure of personal information by an individual to a trusted advisor. The intent of the privilege is to ensure that transfer of information from an individual to his advisor is *not* subject to the ordinary and usual rules of law. The privilege is based on the special nature of the relationship between the communicating parties. Privilege has traditionally been considered a way for an individual to seek aid and support for difficulties of the body, the soul, or the conscience. At their origin, privileged relationships were intended to allow a person to set himself straight with God and man without interference. The clergy, physicians, and attorneys have long been the principal professionals granted this privilege. They are sworn not to disclose what they learn within the scope of working with those who entrust their personal secrets and burdens to them.

As clear-cut as privileged communication would seem to be on its face, it is a concept that is honeycombed with *exceptions*. Those exceptions have created a great deal of misunderstanding and concern among those whose interactions are normally considered privileged. In recent times, a number of legal decisions have held health care providers liable for the wrongful acts of a patient/client because of specific knowledge that a provider had acquired regarding threats of real harm to third parties. In those cases, if the information was not communicated to the appropriate authorities, liability based on a *"failure to warn"* theory was incurred. In other words, *privilege cannot be used as a defense if the life or limb of a third party is endangered.* Our courts have identified, as a matter of "public policy," a *legal duty* that requires health care providers to warn others of perceived harm. This creates a remarkable quandary for the ethical practitioner, for, should he report a threat that does not materialize, he may be guilty of breaching his oath of confidentiality and he may be defaming his patient.

The legal duty to warn is intimately entwined with the judgment of the professional involved. If he perceives real and not improbable lethal danger to a third party, he has, according to several jurisdictions, a legal duty to warn the individual at risk of the harm and is immune from prosecution. If no specific victim is identified, the appropriate authorities should be informed of the risk to unspecified victims. This may be the situation in the case in which a patient with poorly controlled epilepsy refuses to stop driving despite incapacitating seizures or in which a patient with greatly impaired vision similarly refuses not to drive. In general, the less specific the threat or the victim, the less stringent is the duty to warn. This is logical, because public policy is to protect specifically identifiable third parties from harm.

This particular type of privileged communication case has not been tried in many states. The issues will probably be argued, as they have in the past, on the basis of public and state interests in protecting potential victims from harm, versus the right of dangerous individuals to confidentiality because of privileged communication. In some respects, the argument has already been decided in favor of state interests in maintaining law and order and in dealing with protected parties and the public health. For example, physicians are already required by statute to report suspected or actual felonies; the reporting of suspected child abuse to appropriate officials is also law, and there are a substantial number of communicable diseases that physicians must report. It is clear that privileged communications, although generally respected, do have limitations of scope based on public health and general safety considerations of individuals at risk of violence.

It must be emphasized that despite the exceptions noted in privileged communication, the patient generally has the right to have medical communication held in strict confidence. If a physician or his employee discloses confidential information regarding a patient, the physician may be subject to claims of *invasion of privacy; slander;* if the information is negative and conveyed orally; or *libel*, if injurious statements are written. Private communication may be disclosed to third parties only if the patient has granted the physician authority to do so. That authority is most commonly granted in order to provide insurance companies with underwriting data. In some, but not all, states there is automatic waiver of confidentiality regarding conveying information about a patient to a spouse unless the patient specifically denies the waiver. It is a good idea to be familiar with the statutes of your state in this regard.

Physicians frequently express confusion and concern about the release of records to third parties in cases in which their patients have become involved in litigation or quasi-judicial administrative procedures, such as worker's compensation. Under these circumstances, if the matter of health is concerned and the patient's records are to be used as evidence, relevant parts of the record may become subject to discovery. Because the information in the record was provided by the patient with the understanding of confidentiality, physician/patient privilege applies. In some cases, when a patient becomes involved in litigation, the patient's right to certain privileged communication may be waived by a specific state statute. It is suggested that you discuss this matter with your personal legal counsel when you receive requests for information about a patient from state agencies, prosecutors, insurance companies, etc. without an accompanying signed authorization from the patient.

This area of law is very confusing, so it is prudent for a physician who has records subpoenaed or requested, for any reason, to seek immediate legal counsel so that the scope of what is required by a court can be clearly understood. It is important that the physician, as the patient's advocate, protect the privacy of his or her patient and not allow confidential information to get into unauthorized hands.

Special Confidentiality Issues

The coming of the electronic age to medical records is a mixed blessing. It is raising many questions regarding how health care information is stored; how, why, and by whom it may be retrieved; and who may have access to it and for what purposes. In November 1999, the Department of Health and Human Services published a *Notice on Proposed Rule Making* for "Standards for Privacy of Individually Identifiable Health Information" (45 C.F.R. Parts 160-164) based on the requirements of the Health Insurance Portability and Accountability Act of 1996. The objective of the legislation is to protect the privacy of individually identifiable health information that is electronically transmitted. The rules will undoubtedly have immediate and long-term effects on federal and state confidentiality legislation. It is particularly prudent at this time for every physician to review these issues with his or her staff and colleagues, because the field is changing fast and the repercussions are great.

The "confidentiality doctrine," as we stated above, is a privilege between a physician and his or her patient. The confidentiality privilege is based on the need for full disclosure between patient and physician in matters of health care. High-quality care depends on full disclosure. The privilege can be waived *only* by the patient. Therefore, unless there is a written waiver or an authorization in the physician's file, we urge the physician to neither speak nor write outside the medical record about any encounter with a patient. To do so is a breach of confidentiality and subjects the physician to liability should any harm arise to the patient from an unauthorized disclosure. We strongly encourage our readers to become familiar with state laws dealing with medical confidentiality. Circumstances that would ordinarily seem innocuous and proper, such as advising a husband of a wife's health care, or a mother about her teen-age daughter's physical examination, may be fraught with liability, depending on the laws in the jurisdiction in which the physician practices.

Mutual Waivers

In some jurisdictions there are statutory marital waivers regarding health care information for spouses. In those jurisdictions, a physician may freely discuss health care findings and conclusions regarding the health care of a spouse without specific authorization to do so, but waivers for spousal medical care are not the rule across the country. Most jurisdictions would deem such a discussion between a doctor and the spouse of his or her patient a breach of confidentiality of the patient spouse being discussed. On the other hand, if a spouse accompanies the other to the examining room, the physician can be assured that the spouse being evaluated has waived the privilege of confidentiality as it relates to that particular visit. A physician must use sensitivity and judgment in what is said about a patient to anyone, including family, friends, and other interested parties. It is wise to ascertain from the patient just what may be related to others about his or medical circumstances if he or she is hospitalized, incapacitated, or incompetent.

Emancipated Minors

The same is true in dealing with minors who are identified by law as "emancipated minors." Emancipated minors are considered to be adults by the very nature of their personal circumstances. Emancipated minors are individuals, younger than 18, who are *not* under the direct protection and control of parents or guardians. They may be, for example, in the military service or have left home for other reasons and are clearly responsible for their own support and decisions. Unmarried minor mothers are often considered to be emancipated, even if they reside with their parents, because of their specific maternal responsibilities and authority in the care of their child or children.

Mature Minors

Some states recognize another class of minors to whom personal privacy in health care is granted. That group is designated "mature minors." Their privacy is based on the capacity to give a proper informed consent that would be equivalent to that given by a competent adult. The ability to give a proper informed consent is the basis on which this privilege is granted. As we have said elsewhere, a minor may give consent in a life-threatening emergency, but what is more commonly encountered by physicians is the minor teenager who requests confidentiality when he presents himself for care that he does not want disclosed to parents or guardians. The more frequent medical encounter is with young females seeking birth control medications or other contraceptive devices, and boys and girls are frequently seen for care related to sexually transmitted diseases or testing for HIV. A number of states provide statutory support for preserving that confidence, but, in such cases, the minor's parents may not be required to pay the bills incurred, despite the physician's services having been rendered.

The mature minor doctrine does not exist in every state and is usually limited to a circumscribed group of minors who are at least 14 or 15 years of age. In these cases, it is the responsibility of the treating physician to determine whether the child is capable of giving the same type of informed consent as a competent adult would. Thus, the mature minor doctrine does not extend to all minors and depends on the *subjective determination* of the treating physician. In these cases, it is wise for physicians to have legal consultation if there is any question at all as to whether care should be provided to these children without the knowledge and consent of their parents. This is particularly true if an elective surgical procedure is requested by a minor who asks that the care not be divulged by the physician to parents or guardians.

Physicians who treat mature minors and observe the privilege of confidentiality should make note, in their records, of the competency of the children to make health care decisions. It is wise to record something in the nature of "the child requested confidentiality for this care and understood clearly the risks, benefits, and alternatives to this procedure."

HIV and AIDS

Physicians probably don't need reminding about confidentiality related to HIV, AIDS, or genetic testing, but we again remind physicians that, if he or she or staff discloses information related to these topics without a signed authorization from the patient, the doctor may well be liable for any injuries that result.

Consultations and Referrals

Consultations—Are You Exposed

Many physicians wrongly believe that there is little exposure to a malpractice claim when their role is that of a consultant. They believe that the primary physician maintains overall responsibility for the patient. This concept is erroneous. In general, the specialist's role is to deal with that aspect of the patient's care that conforms to his specialty. The consultant has a duty to perform to the standard of care of his specialty. This becomes especially important if the consultant's education and training fall short of the full specialty education. For example, an internist may practice in the area of pulmonary medicine but may not be subspecialty qualified. Any physician that holds him- or herself out as a subspecialist, whether board qualified or not, is held to the performance level as a fully board-qualified subspecialist. Because a referring physician has the right to "act in reliance" based on a specialist's expressed expertise, the consultant, by holding him- or herself out as a specialist in that area of practice, may become a target of litigation if something bad happens to a patient. In their own defense, treating physicians often testify that they relied on a specialist's expertise in the care and treatment of a patient. A common example of this reliance occurs in the field of radiology, where a frequent defense is "I relied on the radiologist."

Although a primary physician may, in good faith rely on the advice of a consultant, some caveats must be considered. If, for example, a primary care physician is perceived to have reviewed an MRI or a CT scan on his own and acts on that review, he will be held to the standard of a radiologist. He cannot claim a lack of training or failure of consultation. On the other hand, we suggest that, when the primary care physician reviews films with a radiologist that he or she note in the patient's chart that the film was reviewed with the radiologist who interpreted the film. The primary physician may add that he concurred with the diagnosis, but the point was that he or she was "acting in reliance" with the interpretation of an expert in that specialty. In this example there is a shared responsibility for an accurate diagnosis, primary care physician and radiologist. The prudent radiologist interprets the film, giving his or her impression and possible alternatives, but allows the clinician to make the diagnosis on the basis of the patient's history and physical findings.

Case Example

A patient was taken to an emergency department with a history of a seizure just prior to his being transported to the ED. A neurologist was called and requested a CT scan of the head and the scan was immediately performed on the patient. The family gave the ED physician a history of head trauma two weeks before the seizure event. The radiologic report noted cerebral edema consistent with head trauma. The radiologist did not note that a cerebral infarct or tumor could not be ruled out from the studies performed. Repeat studies were recommended in four months. The patient's clinical status deteriorated during these four months and follow up studies read by the same radiologist were reported as "no change." The neurologist and the radiologist reviewed the follow-up films together. The treating neurologist relied on the radiologist's report and continued to treat the patient for the seizure disorder for two years. The patient was subsequently worked up by another neurologist, had MRI studies at another institution, and was found to have a malignant brain tumor that was identified as being visible on the prior studies. Both the neurologist and the radiologist were sued for malpractice based on their participation in the patient's care. The neurologist was sued for his failure to ascertain the cause for the progressive deterioration of his patient and the radiologist for his failure to determine that there was a possibility that his symptoms could be due to a tumor or cerebral infarct. The case was settled on behalf of both specialists without a trial.

Hospital and Office Consultations

Specialists called as consults in a hospital setting are required to produce thorough consultation notes. These notes must be accurate and reflect discussions with other physicians, as well as clinical findings and opinions. A well-thought-out differential diagnosis must be set out in the note.

In the case of consultations in an office setting, it is wise to specify the nature of clinical data or laboratory results that were provided by the referring physician. The consultation report should be as complete and accurate as circumstances allow and be placed in the mail or electronically transferred to the referring physician as soon as possible. In emergency circumstances, a call to the referring physician is a good practice. A note in the patient's chart indicating the nature of the call is also wise.

The referring physician has a duty to choose a competent specialist for his or her patient, whether it be for consultation or referral. The primary physician should note in the chart or in the hospital record the reason for the request and note all discussions with the specialist. If films are reviewed with a radiologist, note the gist of the conversations in the chart and record. A note such as "reviewed films with the radiologist" may be insufficient to establish reason for clinical reliance on the opinions or suggestions rendered by the radiologist. On the other hand, if the dated note says, "reviewed the patient's films with the (named) radiologist and reviewed the films. The radiologist felt that this represented an area of swelling in the brain secondary to trauma. No space-occupying lesions observed. I concur with these observations." This notation will help to establish reliance on expert opinion should a legal defense become necessary at a future time.

Area of Concern: Reliance on a Consultant's Advice

Because the law is ever-changing, we want to alert you to an area of concern. This involves on-call, off-the-cuff telephone consultations. We are aware of a case in which a patient went to the emergency department with complaints of chest pain. After a work up, including an ECG, enzymes, and chest x-ray, the ED doctor called the on-call cardiologist to discuss the patient's condition. The cardiologist recommended a second ECG, which was done and was read by the ED doctor as normal. The cardiologist was again called. The ED doctor was advised to proceed with further work up on the patient and call back if needed. Instead of pursuing the cardiologists advice, the ED doctor contacted another on-call internist who suggested a trial of therapy with a GI cocktail and to call back if needed. The patient's symptoms improved after the GI cocktail. The ED physician contacted the patient's family doctor, who agreed to see the patient the next morning. The patient was discharged and died at home later that day of a ruptured aortic aneurysm after his wife left for work.

A suit for medical malpractice was filed and included the ED physician, the cardiologist, the internist, and the hospital. The cardiologist was initially dismissed from the trial on a *directed verdict motion*, but that decision was reversed when the Ohio 12th District Court of Appeals ruled, in essence, that a jury question arose as to whether the cardiologist had acted as a consultant. The court gave a three-part test to be applied:

- Did the doctor participate in making a diagnosis?
- Did he prescribe a course of treatment?
- Did he have a duty to the hospital, the medical staff, and the patient for whose benefit the doctor was in court?

The court of appeals held that a physician-patient relationship can exist by implication when an emergency physician consults with an on-call colleague and the above criteria are met. This case reveals how easy it is to be exposed to medical malpractice litigation. If the cardiologist had requested a fax copy of the ECG (or in other cases an x-ray, blood test results), this behavior would make it clear that liability exposure would exist. This points out that, even without the receipt of records, a consultant has legal exposure in cases of consultation if the requesting doctor relies on the expertise of the consultant in determining the course of the patient's care and the consultant could reasonably deduce that his thoughts or advice would be followed.

Can a discussion in the doctor's lounge or in the hospital hall produce liability? We don't know the answer at this time. It seems that a question such as "what do you think" invokes little potential liability. When the question becomes "what would you do," the potential risk increases. When the weight of a question goes from conceptual inquiry to reliance on process, the risks change.

For physicians who confer over the phone, especially with an emergency department, we recommend that copies of any records received be kept for at least two years and that notes of conversations be placed in a notebook or be tape recorded. In the above example, the cardiologist had little recollection of the call that exposed him to legal liability.

Referrals

Health care providers have a duty to refer patients to other care providers skilled in the area of the patient's need when the condition of a patient is beyond their experience and competence. A dentist discovered gingivitis and suggested to the patient that he go to a specialist because the dentist felt that he wasn't competent to treat the patient's condition, which wasn't responding to his care. At that point, the dentist met the standard. The dentist later testified that the patient, however, balked at the referral and requested that the dentist continue to treat him. The dentist did so without a written consent/waiver and complications arose. The dentist was subsequently sued and lost at trial because his treatment had been inadequate for the condition and failed to meet the standard of care expected of a specialist in that area of dentistry. The point is clear: Refer when in doubt about your care and you will probably be okay, provided the referral is timely and made to a competent specialist. It is perilous to treat a patient beyond your professional competence without a written consent stating the particulars and signed by the patient.

A good practice in patient referrals is to call the consultant and discuss the referral. If the consultant accepts the referral and the patient agrees, obtain an authorization from the patient and copy all or that part of the chart that the referral physician requests, then transfer the records promptly.

The Medical Record

The Hospital Record

In every hospitalization, the medical record includes notations made by any number of care providers. The record should be complete and relevant. It should include a thorough history and physical examination plus all of the laboratory results and notes made by nurses and ancillary personnel. The hospital record, as in the case of the office chart and other medical records, will be taken as gospel at a trial and will be assumed by the experts who review it to be accurate. The hospital record will be used in determining whether the standard of care has been violated. This being the case, it is incumbent on the prudent physician to be certain that all records are clear, concise, and legible. We urge physicians to read nurses' notes, other physician's notes, and any notations made by students. All of these notes may influence a jury; what *you don't know in the hospital record can hurt you*.

A number of cases that have arisen in hospital settings involved the interplay between physicians and nurses. One will frequently see a nurses' note that states something akin to the following: "3:15 a.m. Doctor X notified of patient's condition." At trial, the nurse will testify that the note, though nonspecific, reminds her that she reported everything about the patient's condition to the doctor. On the other hand, the doctor will testify that if he had been told everything, he would have given specific orders to meet the patient's needs or gone to the hospital to see the patient. To avoid this type of finger-pointing dilemma, we recommend that every physician keep a notebook at home and make notes of all patient-related conversations with nurses and others, including the date and time. The notebook can be used as your record of interactions with other professionals in patient care.

Another area of concern is the responsibility of the attending physician to be aware of the patient's condition. With the decrease in the number of nurses, the increase in ancillary personnel, and the increase in each employee's patient load, it will not be sufficient to simply discuss the patient's status with the charge nurse without looking at the nurses' notes. It is recommended that each physician make a notation in the chart that he or she not only spoke with the charge nurse but also reviewed the nursing notes, on a daily basis.

When clinical tests are ordered subsequent to the suggestion or the opinion of another professional, such as a pathologist, a radiologist, or another specialist, it is prudent to note the conversations and the clinical discussion. Colleagues influence the care provided to a patient, so it is good practice to note exactly how that information was acquired and used in formulating the care plan.

If, in reviewing transcriptions, orders, or other chart entries, an error is discovered, it is appropriate to make corrections. The thing is to do it appropriately. In correcting chart notations, create an addendum. Identify the specific error and the correction, and make sure that the addendum is dated and that the time is specified. *Do not correct records after a lawsuit has been filed.* That has the smell of concealment of a problem. This is illegal and will cause no end of grief. If there is an error in a written record, strike out the erroneous item with a single line. Write the correction above the stricken words and initial and date the correction. Again, do not make corrections if a legal case is pending. In a case against a hospital, a resident testified that he realized that a couple of items in the medical record were in error, so he struck out two clauses on the chart and wrote the correction above the errors. The corrections were not dated or timed, and it seemed to a jury that they were added after the patient had experienced complications. The corrections appeared to be an effort to save his backside. The problem was that the doctor wrote the corrections with two different pens in different colors. The jury didn't believe him. Surprise! In another case, a physician had a perfectly neat office chart that was not discolored or smudged, nor did it appear used, although it was alleged to be the record of months of encounters. The case was settled by the physician to avoid a charge to the jury for punitive damages based on tampering with the record.

As stated elsewhere in this book, if you make a mistake, own up to it, tell the patient of the consequences of the error and provide corrective options. Follow up with suggestions for alternative care and call your insurance carrier. That is why you purchase liability insurance. Patients respect personal integrity and concerned care. There was a case some years ago in which a doctor made a mistake during a surgical procedure. He admitted his error and arranged for the patient to be flown, immediately, for care by a recognized specialist in another area of the country. The care was good, and the patient had a good recovery. The patient and the family thanked the initial doctor for his care. Everyone makes mistakes, and usually patients understand when they are told the truth early and earnestly. If one lies, avoids contact with the patient or family, or alters the record and gets caught, he will lose in court and can have punitive damages assessed. Punitive damages are not covered by medical liability insurance.

The Office Chart

Although the patient's chart is technically the physician's property, the patient has a personal and legal interest in the chart, so it is a good practice to act as if it does belong to the patient. With this in mind, the physician should take care to place things in the record as he or she would want to have them seen in the chart by a jury. In our mobile society, people move and change doctors and insurance companies from time to time. It is essential that the record not be tainted by negative personal comments or irrelevant data. The golden rule is a good guideline to use in medical record keeping.

Whether you dictate chart notes for transcription, write notes in the chart or generate your charts electronically, we recommend that all form of notations be completed while the patient is being seen or immediately after seeing the patient. This is a prudent thing to do because at that time your memory of the encounter will be at its absolute best. However it is done, the finished transcript should be carefully read and initialed by you if accurate. If there are errors in the transcription, put a single line through any errors, hand write corrections above the errors, and date and initial the corrections. This is preferred to recreating the chart because it is easily explained and believed. The main thing to remember is *not to make corrections if litigation comes into question.*

If you hand write in your charts, make certain that your notations are legible. Commonly used abbreviations are acceptable. It is sometimes difficult to explain an error in a handwritten chart notation, but when they occur, follow the advice about corrections in the prior section of this chapter. You should use a consistent format in producing chart notes. There are dictionaries of acceptable medical abbreviations. Identify one and stick to the format.

If it is your practice to have a nurse or receptionist write on the chart prior to the physician seeing the patient, be sure to review those notations. If the nurse takes or updates patients' histories, review the updates with the patient and make a notation in the chart regarding the history such as "hx as above", or "hx as above with the additional co/s.o.b. at times." This makes it clear that you reviewed the nurse's notes and talked to the patient about the problem. It is very impressive to see this in writing when defending a physician.

Make certain that all of the physicians that share a practice use the same terminology, abbreviations, and reference points in their notations. Although it didn't make any difference in the legal outcome, a gynecologist was highly embarrassed when she didn't know how to interpret what a partner was referring to when the partner wrote in the chart "8 cm. above the pubic ramus." The physician was not aware of the associate's measuring system and didn't understand his thoughts about the pregnancy at the time of his examination. Fetal age was an issue in that particular case.

Review the chart before seeing a patient. A problem list is a very good summary tool as charts get large. There have been bad results for defendants in more than a few malpractice cases when a doctor failed to look at prior pages of the medical record and thus failed to pursue a problem that had been evident on previous examination. At a trial, a physician simply cannot explain away the failure to be familiar with a patient's chart.

It is good medical practice to have all medically related documents either time stamped or initialed and dated when they arrive at your office. This practice should apply to all correspondence and anything that refers to patient care. If immediate action is required by the information contained in a report, the office record should reflect the action taken and why it was taken. The office record should also reflect telephone contacts with patients. The easiest way to accomplish this is to have a note of each conversation that reflects the patient's current health, any prescriptions, current complaints, etc. A note should be placed in the chart by the individual who spoke to the patient. These notes should also be dated and initialed.

Employee turnover makes it imperative that every entry in a patient's chart be initialed and dated. This makes it much easier to identify potential witnesses to an office event should that become necessary.

Although we have repeatedly cautioned you elsewhere in this book, we caution you one more time, *do not make any changes, corrections, or other notations in a patient's chart,* once any question of litigation arises. At that point, make a copy of the chart for daily use and keep the original chart in a locked, safe place.

If you do locum tenens work or cover a practice for another physician, you need to establish which patients receive routine care and which might have special problems. The charts of patients with special problems should be immediately available to you should problems arise. When you do see a patient of the physician for whom you are covering, you should make a complete record of the interaction. Place the original notations in the office chart and make a duplicate for your own records or those of the agency that schedules your work schedule. While covering a practice for a physician, you should know where and how to contact the physician on whose behalf you are working and contact him or her if there are significant patient care concerns. You should have an emergency plan for any difficulties that occur. Remember, if you assume the care of a difficult patient on your own, you must be willing to bear the responsibility.

Four general rules for good medical record keeping in office, hospital, or other care environments:

1. Stay on topic. Do not digress. Be concise. Be certain that the data are clear, legible, and understandable.

2. Never place anything derogatory in any record. That includes abbreviations that might be interpreted as unflattering or derogatory to a patient. Remember, patients and their attorneys have the right of access to all medical records.

3. Avoid speculation in structuring a clinical work up. Base it on a sound differential diagnosis. Include all clinical findings, laboratory, radiographic and other advanced technical studies as well as all consultations.

4. Be aware of all notations on the record that are not entered by the responsible party—the physician. Read the nurse's notes and those of other care and service providers carefully. Physician defendants have lost in court because of the statements of well-meaning but uninformed persons who have seen fit to interject their views in the record. Juries sometimes do not understand that subtlety.

Part IV

Litigation

This is a rather lengthy segment of the book, and we want you to understand that, because many important legal issues are covered, there will be repetition of essential legal points. The repetitions will help you to understand the ideas and the language of the legal process.

The Initial Stages

Claims and Defenses—How Cases Arise

Establishing the Plaintiff's Case

Because there are a large number of medical malpractice cases around the country, it is not possible to identify a single cause for the many claims. Among the common reasons given by plaintiffs are poor operative or therapeutic results, unexpected injury, death, or expressed dissatisfaction with the care rendered by a physician. With the many advances in medicine over the past several decades and the sensational coverage of those advances by news media, many patients have very high, even unrealistic, expectations of medical and surgical treatments. Anything less than the fulfillment of those expectations can give rise to a legal claim. Unfortunately, not uncommon sources of claims come from the mouths of other physicians who may be critical of a prior treatment. In general, bad or unexpected results of treatment and perceptions of physician indifference are the main causes of malpractice claims.

When patients feel that their care has been inappropriate, many seek legal advice. Attorneys that specialize in representing plaintiffs explore with the patient the nature of the claimed injury and the reasons for the patient wishing to file a claim of wrongful conduct by the physician(s) involved. If there is a significant injury and a probability that the physician(s) involved breached the duty to perform within the standard of care, the discussion will continue. Because of the substantial costs of litigating malpractice cases (e.g., costs of filing a suit, costs of depositions, and expert witness fees), cases in which the damages (monetary compensation paid by the defendant should the plaintiff succeed in winning an award of damages) are likely to be low are generally not pursued. This is not because a small damages case lacks merit but because the economics of litigation make the case a monetary loss for both plaintiff and his or her attorney. When an injury is significant and there is a likelihood of substantial damages, the plaintiff's attorney's interest is piqued. In anticipation of a large verdict or settlement, the patient signs legal authorization that allows the attorney to begin investigating the claim. The establishment of a malpractice claim has two distinct and separate phases as far as a plaintiff's attorney is concerned. The first phase is to determine if a case has legal merit, and the second phase is to determine if the claim will be pursued based on the strength of the available evidence and extent of the damages.

If there is a potential claim, the attorney will write letters to the treating physicians and to the hospital, if hospitalization was involved in the purported injury claim, to ask for copies of the patient's records. When these records are provided, they are reviewed by the attorney and his staff. The staff frequently includes a former nurse or other health care provider. If the records fail to reveal evidence of malpractice, most experienced lawyers will reject the claim and notify the client that there does not appear to be a basis for pursuing the case. This occurs in nearly 90 percent of cases. That generally stops most patients from pursuing litigation. If, on the other hand, a potential claim is recognized by the attorney, the next step is to have the records reviewed by an expert witness.

The Expert Witness

In order to pursue a malpractice claim, a violation of the standard of medical care needs to be established. That step requires that an expert witness be acquired by the plaintiff's attorney. Obtaining an expert witness is not as difficult as some physicians believe. There are many physicians who are quite comfortable looking at claims from a patient's perspective. Many physicians who participate as expert witnesses feel that they play an important role in improving the quality of medical care in general. Most do not act as experts in their own communities because of potential conflicts of interest and/or political clashes. Attorneys often select their experts from a cadre of doctors who have worked with them previously or from published malpractice case reports that list witnesses that have testified at other trials. There are also malpractice witness services that advertise in legal journals. These services list the names of physicians who are willing to review cases for a set fee. Finally, the plaintiff's bar shares experts, via word of mouth, who have proven to be capable witnesses in similar cases.

After reviewing the plaintiff's medical records, the expert witness will contact plaintiff's counsel to give an oral opinion on the merits of the case. If the expert feels that the standard of care was met, the case is generally dropped, and the client is notified that the basis for a malpractice case does not exist and the case should not be pursued. If the expert feels that there has been malpractice but that the outcome would have been, to a high degree of certainty, the same despite medical negligence, the claim will not be pursued. Only when an expert witness opines that the standard of care was violated and that the plaintiff's medical outcome would have been different does the claim continue. This is because the plaintiff has the burden of showing not only that there was malpractice but that the malpractice directly caused serious injury or death.

Filing a Claim or Suit

If the patient's version of the facts, the medical records, and the opinion of one or more expert witnesses support the claim of malpractice, counsel will either make a claim in writing directed to the doctor and/or hospital or file a lawsuit in the court of jurisdiction. The purpose of submitting the claim directly to defendant(s) is to place them on notice of an impending suit in hope of inducing an out-of-court financial settlement. When plaintiff's counsel has plenty of time, settlement negotiations are a reasonable way to proceed, but if plaintiff's counsel is facing a statute of limitations deadline, the suit will be filed immediately to avoid having the case thrown out of court for missing a filing deadline. If the plaintiff's case is very strong, suits are frequently filed before a claim is raised to the defendant. This action puts pressure on the defendant and helps to keep the case moving along. This is a strategy to encourage the defense to expedite a settlement and to prompt the defense to move along in assessing its case. It takes time for the doctor and the insurance company to investigate the merits of the case and the sooner it's settled or litigated, the sooner the plaintiff and the attorney are paid.

Resolution of Claims

Sometimes counsel for the patient/plaintiff will obtain a written report from a medical expert and will send that report along with a letter to the defendant physician and/or hospital, requesting that their insurance carriers or appropriate risk management agents contact plaintiff's counsel to discuss a possible resolution to the claim without having to resort to litigation. If the doctor, hospital, and insurance company feel that a settlement is in order, counsel for the patient/plaintiff will be contacted in order to substantiate the claim. At that point plaintiff's counsel will put together a settlement package that will include copies of the appropriate medical records, copies of billings, cost of follow-up medical care, verification of lost wages, photographs that depict the alleged injury and other documents that support the claim, along with a demand, in dollars, to settle the case. After the insurance company and/or risk manager have investigated the claim, a meeting is scheduled to try to resolve the case. Because of the many complexities in establishing malpractice cases and the time constraints related to filing a case, i.e., statutes of limitations, very few cases are resolved prior to the filing of a lawsuit.

Statute of Limitations

Every malpractice case has to deal with the issue of a state's statute of limitations from the start. The statute of limitations is simply a time limit set by the state legislature on the filing of a legal claim. For example, in Ohio, a malpractice case must be filed within one year of the time that the claim arose, i.e., the time that the injury occurred; or from the time that the claimant discovers through reasonable care and diligence that an injury had occurred, if the injury was not obvious at the time that it occurred. For example, because a patient would have no way of knowing that a sponge left in the operative site during a procedure would subsequently cause complications, courts have felt that to leave a patient without a remedy due to an obvious error was improper. In Ohio, and in most other states, the discovery rule adopted by the courts holds that a cause of action accrues and the statute of limitations begins to run when a reasonably prudent person, in the position of the plaintiff, knew or should have known that he sustained injury as a result of the action or failure of action of a specific physician and/or institution. The rule is applied on a case-by-case basis and is not specifically dependent on exactly when the patient discovered the malpractice. In making this determination the court uses the reasonable man standard to determine when the plaintiff became aware or should have become aware of the extent and seriousness of his condition and whether he was aware that the condition was related to the specific medical service rendered.

If an action is not filed within one year of the occurrence or discovery of negligence, a suit is legally barred from being pursued by the injured party. Every state has legislation setting time limits on the filing of cases, and every physician should learn the applicable period of limitations in his or her state. In wrongful death cases based on medical malpractice, there is a different limitation in Ohio and in some other states. In Ohio that type of claim must be brought forth within two years of the death. A wrongful death based on malpractice occurs when the alleged malpractice directly and proximately caused the death of a patient, whether the death is immediate or delayed.

All statutes of limitation have nuances that are important to be aware of. For example, in Ohio, there is a statute of limitations on what is called a 180 Day Letter. The statute allows for an extension of the statute of limitations that permits the plaintiff's counsel sufficient time to investigate a case when a potential claim is presented just prior to the statutory time limit. The mandated methodology for the submission of a 180 Day Letter is very specific and must be followed precisely in order to gain the extension. The extension of 180 days begins when the letter is delivered to the physician and/or hospital and not 180 days from the date of the patient/plaintiff's last treatment or date of injury.

Statutes of Limitations—Discovery Rule

An extension of the statute of limitations may well occur during the period of discovery by the plaintiff's attorney. The extension is granted in order to allow the plaintiff's attorney to ascertain whether there may have been additional, undiscovered injuries not evident at the time that the claimed injury was caused. Discovery allows the plaintiff to determine whether there might be other medical problems, not previously evident, incurred at the time of the alleged act of medical negligence. A malpractice claim may be broadened when a patient is found to have developed complications or symptoms from, for example, a foreign body, such as a surgical sponge, negligently left in the abdomen When the extension is applicable, the plaintiff can have the period extended by an additional 180 days by simply delivering a 180 Day Letter letter to the defendant. Extension of the statute of limitation is not applicable in wrongful death cases.

An example of the above situation will help to explain the point. Some years ago a case was filed in Ohio by a woman who claimed that a hospital physician committed malpractice. She felt that she had been injured while she was in the hospital so she went to see an attorney. After a short conference with the attorney, she was told that she didn't have a case, so she went on her way. Months later her condition worsened and she saw another attorney who filed suit more than one year after she had seen the first lawyer. A defense motion for summary judgment was filed after the woman was deposed, the court held that the suit was time barred, because the woman suspected, when she saw the first lawyer, that she had a potential claim. The first attorney was then sued for malpractice for having failed to file a timely claim. The outcome of that case is unknown to us because it is likely that there was a settlement between the attorney and his client. Settled cases don't get much publicity.

The issue of the statute of limitations arises in every malpractice case and often results in legitimate cases being turned down because the patient didn't seek legal help within the prescribed period. In summary, a plaintiff's case is established for purposes of pursuit when:

- The injury to the patient is significant or death has occurred.
- The medical records support the plaintiff's claim.

- There is an expert or experts in the field willing to testify that a deviation from appropriate care standards occurred and proximately caused significant injury to the plaintiff.

- The statute of limitations has not expired.

Only when these factors are operative does a case proceed. As you can imagine, time, effort, and expense (i.e., costs of obtaining records, fees for expert review, staff and attorney time) are to be carefully considered in a situation in which the odds of the plaintiff's winning the case are approximately one in ten.

Claims Process

If a patient decides to bring a malpractice suit against you, the first notice that you will receive is likely to be a letter from an attorney requesting a copy of the patient's medical records. If you know that the patient has not been injured in an auto accident, at work, or on someone else's property, you should suspect that a possible claim for malpractice is being considered against you. This is particularly true if you have reason to believe that the patient is in any way unhappy with your care. If the letter is accompanied by an authorization signed by the patient that is less than 60 days old, you have an obligation to copy and send to counsel the records requested. What you do from this point on is very important to your long-term legal well-being.

The very first thing you should do when you receive the request is to contact your personal attorney for advice on how to proceed. The rules vary from jurisdiction to jurisdiction, and you want to clearly understand your obligations. Follow your attorney's advice on how to respond and on how much, if anything, to charge for providing the copies. The next call should be to your malpractice insurance carrier to notify the agent of the request for records. This must be done expeditiously for you to comply with policy requirements related to notification of any possible action against you. *The next thing* that needs to be done is to make two copies of the patient's medical file. One copy will be provided to the requesting attorney and the second copy will be used as a substitute for the original in your office file. The original record should be kept in a secure place, such as a safe box or locked file cabinet, until the legal matter is resolved. When the matter is resolved, you can place the original record in the file and discard the copy. Until that occurs, the original file must be protected from any inadvertent alterations or losses that can occur when a file is used and copied during a malpractice case. Of course, no changes are to be made on the original record after a request for the record by an attorney.

Providing Records to the Plaintiff's Attorney

After the above steps have been taken, write a letter to the requesting attorney stating that a copy of the requested chart is enclosed along with a bill for the expense of copying. Start a new file folder for the patient using the record copy made for that purpose and place a copy of the attorney's letter with the authorization and a copy of your letter in a new and separate "litigation" file. This file will contain any and all pertinent correspondence related to the case should a suit be brought against you. Be sure to follow the advice of your counsel regarding the addition of notes to the "litigation" file. Notes that you add to the file may reflect such things as your personal recollections of the patient and your thought processes in treating the patient. As indicated in other portions of this book, these notes and written reflections about the case are protected from discovery by the attorney-client privilege if done at the specific direction of your lawyer. Once the file is created, you need do nothing else, as the matter will now be handled by your attorney and the insurance company. *Do not, under any circumstances, make further contact with the plaintiff's lawyer.* Do not talk to him on the phone, do not meet with him, and do not write to him. No good can come from talking to him. If you are curious about the nature of a possible claim, your attorney can investigate for you. The physician may wish to discontinue in the care of the patient at this point. If so, send a letter of withdrawal from the case to the patient. Advise the patent to seek other qualified care givers and provide a date of termination which allows the patient reasonable time to find a physician. Some physicians choose to continue care even under these circumstances. Either choice is a matter to be discussed with legal counsel.

Suit is Filed – What Do I Do Now

If a lawsuit is filed, either the Clerk of Courts will send you a summons by mail or the County Sheriff or his designee will personally present these documents to you. A summons is simply the legal way of notifying you that you are being sued and that you have a certain number of days to respond to the suit. The summons will not tell you why you are being sued. The specific allegations against you are found in the complaint, which will spell out in very simple language what the case is all about. How you handle the fact that you are being sued is very important.

Sensitive Mail Policy

In order to avoid the stress of rumors being initiated in an office, there should be an office policy stating that any letters received from lawyers are to be opened only by the physician addressed or by an appointed staff member, usually the practice manager. All such letters must be absolutely private and confidential and not the business of the staff. If a letter deals, in any way, with a possible malpractice case, the policy must be that the letter be immediately placed in the hands of the physician(s) involved. This procedure will protect physician(s) and staff members from later being questioned about discussion of the letter. Discussions related to a malpractice case are not privileged within an office and discussions with staff or associates are discoverable by a plaintiff's attorney. If a suit is filed, the policy must be that all letters from the court, any attorney, or the insurance company must be delivered, unopened, to the physician involved.

When you read a summons and complaint, do so in the privacy of your office or home. Do not talk to anyone about the lawsuit. Your first reaction is not likely to be a favorable one, and you may say something, e.g., to a staff member or associate, that you may later regret. It is permissible, if you feel you must, to notify your staff of the fact that you have been sued and by whom, but any other comments or information would be inappropriate. If other physicians are named in the suit, *do not talk to them about the lawsuit.* We repeat, such conversations are discoverable by the plaintiff's attorneys. If, on the other hand, other physicians named in the suit speak to you, you may *listen*, as they may help you later in your defense, but by no means should you respond or discuss the case. The comments of others can be used by your attorney in preparing your defense but it is important that you not provide another's attorney with materials useful to his or her client(s). *Listen but do not talk.*

The Insurance Company Lawyer

When you are contacted by the lawyer hired by your professional liability insurance company to represent you in the litigation, you have a duty to cooperate completely. Advise him or her that you have a personal lawyer and what you have done up to that point on advice of counsel. You will be working with both lawyers from this time on, but remember that the insurance company is footing the bill for your defense, so we suggest that you allow the insurance lawyer to clearly take the lead in organizing the defense. Your personal counsel is involved as a sideline advisor to protect matters of personal interests. Experienced lawyers know how to interact in these matters, and it is best to follow their advice. Work with the insurance counsel and keep your own attorney apprised of any concerns that you may have. If you are not satisfied for any reason with the insurance company lawyer, speak directly with your personal lawyer, with whom you should have already discussed your concerns. You may also express any concerns to your insurance agent.

Policy Limits

Another thing that you will want to do when a suit has been filed is to ascertain from your insurance agent, personal lawyer, and defense counsel the policy limits (dollar limits) that apply to the suit filed against you. If the claim exceeds your policy limits, there is a potential for personal financial exposure that must be considered. This is why we emphasize that before you are exposed to litigation, you should seek legal advice from your personal lawyer as to the best means of protecting your assets. He may recommend another lawyer who specializes in asset protection to help you. Remember, if you do not have a comprehensive estate plan and you are sued, your personal assets may well be in jeopardy. Be sure that you are adequately insured so that your personal assets are well protected. We strongly recommend that you contact your professional liability insurance agent and personal attorney as soon as possible to deal with all of these issues.

You should know whether your malpractice policy requires your consent to settle a claim or suit. Some professional liability policies leave settlement solely up to the discretion of the company. If your policy does, you will want to start thinking about how that provision could affect you should you be sued. You will also want to check, from time to time, on the financial health of your malpractice carrier. The insurance commissioner's office of your state can advise you. Don't choose a carrier strictly on the basis of lower rates. Choose a malpractice carrier of strong reputation that has been and will likely be in business in the long-term future.

Structuring the Defense

Good News

Most malpractice cases tried in this country result in verdicts in favor of physicians and/

or hospitals. Even so, it is unwise to become complacent about the defense of a case. Although statistics favor the defense, we have seen defensible cases lost because of a failure to properly prepare the defense and/or to be prepared for trial. Plaintiffs usually win the very solid cases in which malpractice is clear. Those cases are generally settled prior to trial. The defendants win the remainder, barring, of course, the occasional unexplainable jury verdict.

After notifying your attorney and the insurance carrier and setting up a personal litigation file as directed by your counsel, you will want to meet with the attorney assigned to your defense by the insurance company. It is important that you understand that it is the assigned lawyer's responsibility to protect your interests, to represent you in court, and to file various pleadings on your behalf. Notify your personal counsel of the insurance company's selection and the date that you will first meet with your counsel.

The first meeting with the assigned attorney is very important. You will want to bring with you the entire patient's chart, with complete copy for the attorney. It is important that you are working together from the same exact record. You will want to explain, in detail, what the record says and what it means. Provide full disclosure, good or bad. Be candid with counsel about the case as you know it. Don't be afraid to express your feelings and concerns at this meeting. Inform counsel of any persons with whom you may have spoken about the case and try to recall exactly what was said. Be prepared to give counsel the names, addresses, and phone numbers of employees from your office who have had contact with the patient or who have made entries on the patient's chart. You should also discuss any thoughts or notions made in your private litigation file, as the confidentiality doctrine also applies to this attorney. Discuss the case until you feel that counsel fully understands the case from your perspective.

It is important to understand that, from this point forward, your role is to be a witness in the litigation. The legal aspects of your defense are the responsibility of your counsel. It is very important that you have confidence in your attorney. You want to feel that he or she understands the facts of the case and feels that the case can be defended. You want to feel confident that you have an able ally representing you. The assigned counsel will try the case while your personal counsel will remain out of the limelight to protect your personal interests. Both have important roles in your defense.

During the initial visit, you will want to discuss with counsel the nature of the plaintiff's claim and begin to plan a defense. You will want to know if the suit has been filed in a timely manner and whether there are expert witness reports that are critical of you. If your first knowledge of a claim was the filing of a lawsuit, your counsel may have little information available from the other side. This should not be of concern to you, as all states require full disclosure to defendants. Your counsel, with the use of discovery, will obtain all the relevant medical documents and opinions of opposition expert witnesses in due time.

You will want to ask counsel how you can help in the early stages of the process. If the issue includes procedures that involve medical expertise, you may be asked to conduct some medical literature research under counsel's direction. Counsel may also want to discuss with you potential expert witnesses who will look at the case from your perspective. You will not want to use close friends or colleagues as witnesses, nor will you want to ask former teachers, even if they are experts in the field in question. This is a case where their credibility would be suspect because of the established relationship with them. The role of expert witnesses is to be objective about the issues in question. Anything that taints objectivity affects credibility. *Do not be concerned if you cannot identify an expert yourself.* Your attorney has many sources for finding experts, including other defense attorneys and doctors known to your insurance company. You may want to consider seminar speakers who are respected for their expertise in the area in question.

Staying Informed

You should also discuss with counsel your role in the ensuing months. You may request that counsel provide you with copies of all correspondence with opposing counsel or expert witnesses as well as any letters to the insurance carrier pertaining to the case be copied to you. You have a right to know everything that is going on in your case, especially if you have the right of approval of any settlement offered by your insurance company. You will *not* want to receive copies of interrogatories or requests for documents (covered later in this chapter) that are sent by your lawyer to opposing counsel, because they are unanswered questions sent to uncover the basis of the other side's case. You will want to receive copies of the answered interrogatories and answered requests for documents, including all medical records and expert reports that are received by your counsel during discovery. Understanding what is transpiring will allow you to use your medical background to aide counsel in understanding the medical issues gleaned from the records.

Exhibits

You will want to discuss with counsel the use of demonstrative exhibits during trial. These may include x-rays, scale anatomical models, or photographs. You will want to have a time line of events to demonstrate to the jury your involvement in the case and the status of things during your participation. A time line can be a simple graph that demonstrates a sequence of events, patient status, orders, test results, and nursing observations as reflected by the records. Time lines are particularly useful in cases involving long-term hospital cases or cases including the issue of prescription usage over time, such as Coumadin® therapy.

Time lines should be based on the sequence of events recorded in the medical record. For example, a patient was brought to the emergency department with a history of a horse falling on him. Initial x-rays revealed two fractured ribs and a pneumothorax on one side. A surgeon was called and a chest tube was placed. The patient was admitted to the intensive care unit. The surgeon left but called an internist on medical staff call to discuss the case and the patient's status. The patient later began to develop dyspnea, and the internist was called by a nurse. Another chest film and blood gases were ordered by the internist, who said he was on his way. Upon arrival he read the films, which he did not feel were diagnostic of pneumothorax on the opposite side. He went to evaluate the patient, who was at this time stable but who was described as "resembling the Michelin man." The internist called the surgeon to alert him to a possible need for placement of another chest tube. He then ordered another chest film and went to talk to the patient's spouse. At that point the roof caved in. The patient became severely dyspnic and was hardly breathing when the internist was again called by a nurse. He immediately re-evaluated the patient and intubated him. The patient rapidly improved. His blood gases were almost back to normal when the cuff on the endotracheal tube deflated and the tube came out of the trachea. Unfortunately, the patient vomited and aspirated on attempts to re-intubate him. The emergency department doctor was summoned, and a tracheostomy was performed. Valiant efforts were instituted to save the patient, but he expired.

As you can imagine, the widow sued everyone involved. The most confusing issue in the suit was the nurse's notes, which were done on scratch paper while all of these events were going on. The notes were a problem in that they were off in time sequence by approximately an hour from all major events when compared with verifiable times, such as the time of chest films, blood samplings, and physician notations in the chart. The internist's independent memory of the times of the two calls that he received at home also indicated that the nurse's notes were in error. By developing his own time line, he was able to construct a sequence of events that specifically established when he was called, when he arrived at the hospital and the patient's condition when he took over care. It was extremely helpful during depositions of the plaintiff's experts and the defendants to have the sequence of events established, and it also helped to clarify each physician's responsibilities during the course of the evening.

Other useful tools in the defense of malpractice cases are medical illustrations. These are anatomically correct illustrations made by professionals, sometimes with the aid of the defendant physician. The physician can guide the illustrator in modeling the illustration to fit the circumstances of the case. In a case filed against a surgeon for injury to the femoral nerve with electrocautery during an abdominal operation for Crohn's disease, a medical illustration was employed. The basic anatomy of the abdomen and the pelvis were presented with overlays to show the location of the various abdominal and pelvic organs and their relationship to the femoral nerve. This was extremely helpful, because the jury understood that the use of cautery in the upper abdomen was not likely to have caused injury to the femoral nerve, despite the claim of the plaintiff's expert witness.

In our experience, plaintiff's counsel is more likely to use medical illustrations than the defense. Prior to trial you will want to know if the other side will be using them and will want to become familiar with them. It is important that you and your lawyer determine the accuracy, completeness, and relevance of any illustrations. With computers many plaintiffs' lawyers are now constructing visual models demonstrating procedures and techniques based on the operative notes and information gained in depositions to illustrate surgical procedures to juries. It sometimes seems that the plaintiff's bar is a step ahead of the defense bar in the use of technology. The plaintiff's bar is frequently more willing to spend the money necessary to gain an edge with a jury. We must remember that most jury members receive most of their health information from television or computers and tend to believe what they see and hear from those media.

Time lines, medical illustrations, and other visual aids are not necessary in every case. Our recommendation is to consider their use in every case and rule them out as unnecessary rather than using them when their effectiveness might be minimal. A couple of simple questions placed in interrogatories or during the deposition of witnesses will let your attorney know early on whether the plaintiff's side is preparing to use visual aids. Learning of their use in advance of trial is a way to lessen their impact. If they are to be used, plaintiff and defense counsels may agree to the joint use of stipulated exhibits for trial or the defense may, prior to trial, attempt to exclude the illustrations because they are inaccurate, misleading, or incomplete. Dealing with these questions is the responsibility of your counsel, but the better that you understand the legal process the better you are able to assist counsel in providing the best defense possible. The days of trying major and complicated cases with the testimony of witnesses alone are gone. Today visual aids, including excerpts from video depositions are the norm, so work with counsel to be prepared in all facets of defense.

Pre-Trial Motions

A motion is a written request to the court for a ruling on an issue in dispute. These can range from a motion for clarification of the plaintiff's claim against a defendant to a motion for an extension of time to provide an adequate defense or to comply with a prior court order. These motions are handled by counsel and generally will not require your involvement. We do suggest that you ask your insurance company-appointed counsel to copy any motions and responses to your personal attorney and to you. We feel that it is important that you know the precise status, at all times, of the litigation. Review all motions filed. Any questions that you may have regarding these filings should be addressed to insurance counsel.

The most important pretrial motion is a motion for summary judgment. This motion is made in an effort to persuade the court that, even if everything the plaintiff alleges is true, recovery against the defendant would be barred for any number of specific legal reasons, such as failure to file within the statute of limitations or failure to demonstrate a breach of duty. These motions are not filed in every case, but they are appropriate when a plaintiff's case is weak or when the other side has not produced an expert witness. This motion is also appropriate when a claim for punitive damages is made.

A claim for punitive damages is an allegation by the plaintiff that the defendant's conduct was egregious or that the care and treatment of a patient demonstrated total or reckless disregard for his or her rights and well-being. If a summary judgment motion is granted by the court to the defense on the punitive damages claim, that issue is thrown out and the case proceeds only on the malpractice claim. It is important to remember that *punitive damages are not covered by medical malpractice insurance* and that the financial exposure from an award for punitive damages falls fully on the defendant physician. It is therefore important that a summary judgment motion be filed by the defense any time that a claim for punitive damages is made. There are two reasons; first, if the defense prevails, the punitive damages claim will be dismissed; second, if the motion fails, defense counsel will be able to prepare a defense on that claim prior to trial.

When defense counsel files a motion for summary judgment, the defendant may be asked to prepare and sign an affidavit, a written statement made under oath. Since an affidavit is sworn testimony, everything in it can be used in questioning the defendant during deposition and trial. Therefore, it is extremely important that the affidavit be accurate and correct. Do not authorize use of your affidavit if you feel uncomfortable in any way with its content. For example, it would be *appropriate* to sign an affidavit that states that you complied with the standard of care while caring for the plaintiff. It would be *inappropriate* to sign an affidavit that states that you did nothing wrong. Although the differences are subtle, they are important, because, if you should admit to making even a harmless error, the first statement would shield you while the second could be used against you. It is important to work closely with defense counsel in preparing the affidavit. When it is completed, read it carefully. We urge you to also review it with your personal counsel as well, with this thought in mind: "Are there any statements or words in the affidavit that can be used against me?" If the answer is yes, work with counsel and start again.

There are a number of other motions that can be filed and used by defense counsel during the course of litigation prior to trial. These are procedural and technical motions that are used to try to limit the scope of the lawsuit or to have it dismissed. If you have any concerns about these motions, speak with your counsel, but, as a general rule, it is best practice to let your lawyer defend the case while you concentrate on being a good witness.

As mentioned above, a motion for summary judgment is particularly effective when one of the defense claims is that the plaintiff's claim is barred by the statute of limitations. As mentioned above, state laws require that claims for medical malpractice be filed within a certain time limit, usually one year; if the malpractice suit is not filed within the time limit stipulated by statute the entire case will be dismissed. This defense claim must not be overlooked.

The Process of Discovery—Search for the Truth

Discovery in a lawsuit is designed to allow the opposing parties to learn everything that they can about the lawsuit raised. It allows each side to see which cards the other will play in a trial. Among the purposes of discovery is to prevent a "legal ambush" at trial. Discovery allows the attorneys to prepare their pre-trial motions, to limit the scope of claims and defenses to be used in trial. A number of devices are employed by counsel in discovery. The following summary is designed to provide physicians with a basic understanding of the various discovery procedures employed in litigation. The following legal topics will be discussed individually:

- Interrogatories
- Depositions
- Production of documents
- Requests for admissions
- Physical examinations

Interrogatories—Written Questions and Answers

Under the Federal Rules of Civil Procedure, which govern the conduct of all civil actions brought in federal district courts and have been adopted by most state courts, interrogatories are written questions directed to the parties to a lawsuit. These questions must be answered in writing and under oath. There have been numerous judicial decisions dealing with interrogatory questions but it is beyond the scope of this book to discuss them. It is sufficient to say that there are generally accepted rules that are followed in the process of acquiring the requested information. In general, interrogatories are sent to the plaintiffs and defendants to acquire basic information about the principals in the case. Information requested usually pertains to date of birth, social security number, marital status, and educational background. In addition, they are used to learn the identity of fact witnesses, expert witnesses, the location of critical documents and records, the names of physicians currently involved in the care of the plaintiff, the dates and sites of inpatient or outpatient visits, and other information that is relevant to support claims and defenses in a malpractice case. Interrogatories are used by the defense primarily to identify the persons and documents that form the basis of the plaintiff's claim.

The responses to interrogatories are made under oath, just as affidavits are. The answering party swears that the answers are correct and accurate. Answers must be carefully prepared by your attorney with your help, and you must be satisfied with your answers, as they will be the basis for plaintiff's counsel's questions in deposition and at trial. Ideally, the answers to interrogatories should be brief. One must be leery of questions that require lengthy responses because a failure to include some detail could be harmful. In Ohio, for example, an attorney can object to questions that require narrative responses *(Penn Central v. Armco* 56 O 2nd 95). Do *not* agree to any answer that makes you uncomfortable, even if your counsel recommends it. Remember that your lawyer doesn't have to testify regarding the answer, but you will. Read the question carefully and answer truthfully and accurately. After the answers are typed, work with your defense attorney to determine whether:

- There is anything in the responses that can be used against you.

- There is anything that is inaccurate.

- Your response will be the same if the same question is asked in court.

- The answers might be misleading.

- You left something important out of a response.

If you are satisfied with the responses, sign the answers and make sure that you and your personal counsel receive copies. Remember, your answers to interrogatories are admissible as evidence at trial.

Depositions—the Ultimate Weapon

A deposition is a question and answer session conducted under oath with the questions and answers being recorded by a court reporter or a videographer. Again, your answer to every question is evidence that is admissible in a trial court, so the importance of a deposition cannot be overstated. Depositions are the most important events to occur in a malpractice case prior to trial, so we will go into detail on this important topic.

Scheduling

Depositions in a malpractice case are usually scheduled informally by counsel on a date and at a time convenient to the litigants and counsel. Counsels agree on date, time, location, and who will be deposed. Although most depositions are conducted before a court stenographer/ reporter, they may be video recorded. After all of the arrangements are made, a "Notice of Deposition" will be filed with the trial court to inform the court of the proceeding and to formally notify counsel of the commitment.

In some jurisdictions opposing counsel has the authority to serve the defendant and his or her attorney with a filed "Notice of Deposition" that requires the defendant to be at a certain place and time to be deposed. This notice is legally binding. If the defendant receives this type of notice and it creates inconvenience, the defense attorney must be contacted immediately. Defense counsel has legal recourse in dealing with scheduling problems caused by this type of notice.

Location

A physician's deposition may be taken for several reasons. He may be the *plaintiff's physician*. In that case he will be called as a witness of fact to the plaintiff's condition. He will testify only to the current status of the patient. There will be no questions requiring opinions related to the cause of the patient's current circumstances. A physician may also be deposed as an *expert witness*, in which case he will help to define the standard of care and issues of causation related to the plaintiff's claim. If you are to be a witness under either of these circumstances, the best location for the deposition will be your office. This location will save travel and minimizes time away from the office. In addition, you will feel more comfortable in the familiar surroundings.

If you are the defendant in a lawsuit, it is strongly recommended that your deposition be taken at your lawyer's office. Although you may feel more comfortable in your own office, having a deposition there may open the door to certain inquiries that you may not wish to have explored. For example, questions may be raised about billing practices. You may then be asked to produce billing documents, because they are present and available. This may produce information that may be irrelevant to the lawsuit but unfavorable for you (e.g., your description of a procedure for insurance purposes). You may be asked about certain books or treatises that you have in your office and why you keep those handy. Those things could come back to haunt you during cross-examination at trial. You might be asked whether you agree with certain statements taken directly from the books on your shelves. You may have to defend yourself from the implication that you consider the books to be authoritative in their entirety because you keep them as references in your office. We want you to know that you can respond to that type of question by saying that you do not accept any book or article as wholly authoritative. This clearly expresses the feeling that you disagree with the statement, but you may still be subject to the question "then why do you keep that volume on your desk?" This is just one among many reasons that you should not be deposed in your office if you are a defendant.

You will be asked to list the materials that you reviewed to prepare for the deposition and may be asked to produce them. If the materials are in your office, this could prove embarrassing to you and your attorney, particularly if you had not yet fully discussed them with your counsel. There are just too many things that may arise in a deposition conducted in your office that can give aid to opposing counsel. If the deposition is conducted at your attorney's office and you are asked about billings or texts, your attorney can arrange to review with you regarding those requested items and produce or object to their production as your interests dictate at a later date. You can save yourself a lot of distress by going to the attorney's office to be deposed.

The notice of deposition may contain a *duces tecum* notation that specifically identifies certain documents that the other attorney demands that you bring with you to the deposition. This request will usually include the patient's chart, billing records and your personal and office calendar. It is imperative that you get together with your lawyer as soon as you receive the *duces tecum* notice so that you can go over the list of what is requested and identify whether any of the items are legally protected and beyond discovery. Rely on your attorney as to what you must produce at the deposition. It is counsel's responsibility to protect you and to go over each document that you must produce and prepare you as to how to answer questions about each of the items.

In responding to a *duces tecum* notice, take some time to update and correct your curriculum vitae (C.V.). Make sure it is accurate and, by all means, do not inflate or minimize your credentials. Do not put anything in your C.V. that is not specifically accurate. For example, if you have listed attendance at seminars in an area of interest that is usually handled by specialists, you will want to make sure that the C.V. reflects your interest but not a specialist's level of knowledge. Remember, the legal rule related to all physicians is, "If you hold yourself out as a specialist, you will be held to the higher standard required of a specialist." If you are a generalist, make sure that your C.V. accurately reflects that level of background.

If you follow the advice given elsewhere in this book, the patient's chart will be in the same condition that it was the day that you were notified of the claim, with nothing added or deleted. The private "litigation file," which has documents that you filed upon direction of your attorney, need not be produced as it is protected from discovery. The litigation file will also contain correspondence between you and your attorney, or your insurance company. You will want to review the litigation file with defense counsel when preparing for deposition. Counsel can identify the items in the file that you should produce at deposition, such as answers to interrogatories, the initial letter of notice from the plaintiff, and your responses before the suit was filed. After meeting with counsel and determining what is and is not privileged, you can answer questions at deposition about what you may have reviewed prior to the deposition. You do not have to reveal the review of any privileged materials.

Date and Time

It is our opinion that the discovery deposition is the most important pre-trial event in a malpractice case. During a deposition, opposing counsel will try to learn everything that you know about the patient's care and treatment. It is important that you be well rested before a deposition and, although this suggestion may cause office scheduling headaches, we feel that the best time for your deposition is on a Monday morning. The next best times are the days following a day off or the day following a holiday. The absolute worst times are the afternoons following heavy morning schedules or evenings after office hours. The reasons are obvious. No sane physician should want to schedule the most critical aspect of a lawsuit at a time when he or she is fatigued or when other pressing matters have to be dealt with. Clear the day of patient responsibilities and use the weekend or the day before to carefully prepare yourself for the challenge.

Cardinal Rules for Deposition

Below is a list of widely accepted guidelines established by the trial bar for answering questions during depositions. These can be used as your guide in answering deposition questions:

- Answer every question honestly.

- If you don't know the answer, don't be afraid to say so.

- If you don't understand the question, ask that it be repeated or rephrased.

- Answer only the question asked. If you feel the need to explain an answer, give the explanation but be aware of the fact that verbal digressions can create problems by introducing new information into the mix. Remember that your trial attorney can revisit a question asked by plaintiff's counsel if you were not satisfied with your original response. Allow counsel to help you to determine just what you should say.

- Don't guess or speculate in answer to a question.

- Don't get angry or lose your composure.

- The law deals in probabilities not possibilities.

- Be prepared to answer dumb and/or irrelevant questions.

- Don't volunteer information. Digressions are trouble.

- Don't be defensive or argumentative. Juries may view these behaviors as incriminating.

These rules and others will be brought up at length by your attorney. They are presented here simply to guide your thoughts and to prepare you to be deposed.

Depositions—Dress Well But Don't Be Flashy

Among physicians who become defendants in malpractice suits, a frequently asked question is, "How should I dress for the deposition?" If a deposition is to take place in your office, you may wear a lab coat because that is appropriate to the location. We advise against brandishing a stethoscope, because some people consider that to be an affectation. Make sure that the lab coat is clean and neat and that any name or insignia on the coat is consistent with the practice. For male physicians, if you feel better in a suit or sport coat, that is also appropriate but do not wear jeans, an open shirt, or a lot of jewelry. Avoid appearing flashy by brandishing expensive cuff links, rings, and watches. You want to appear confident, successful, and modest, not gaudy. The female practitioner likewise should feel comfortable in a lab coat if the deposition is in her office. A nice dress or a business suit is also appropriate. The dress should always extend below the knee and modest jewelry is appropriate. Any jewelry should lend a touch of class but not appear ostentatious. Gem stones and other expensive jewelry should not be worn. Wedding bands, class rings, and other jewelry that emphasize family or school loyalties are certainly appropriate. If the deposition is to be taken in your lawyer's office, business attire is appropriate for both male and female physicians.

Dress is even more important if the deposition is to be videotaped. At a video deposition the videographer records your responses. Many malpractice attorneys videotape the depositions of a defendant in a lawsuit to get a feel for the credibility of the defendant and to define weaknesses in the testimony that may be reflected in the defendant's demeanor. Facial expressions, uncomfortable pauses, worried looks, or looks away from the camera for assistance are noted as well as the words used. Deposition videotapes are played for other members of the plaintiff attorney's law firm and for sample juries who are paid for by counsel for the plaintiff in order to obtain a sense of how a real jury would respond to the defendant's testimony. The videotapes are also played for jury consultants who suggest the type of juror most likely to be sympathetic or unsympathetic to the plaintiff's cause. They are also shown to expert witnesses hired by the plaintiff's lawyer to testify against the defendant.

Depositions, whether in written or video form, can be used at trial by the plaintiff's attorney to discredit testimony before a jury if something is said that varies from the previously recorded testimony. At times the video is presented as part of the plaintiff's case, particularly if the defendant's deposition revealed uncertainty and anxiety. Juries watch the facial expressions and demeanor of the defendant on the deposition video in addition to listening to his responses to questions. For these reasons personal appearance and demeanor at a deposition are highly important. We encourage defendants to be consistent in their dress. One does not want to appear casually dressed at deposition and well-dressed at trial, because that implies inconsistency in behavior. In all cases, clothing must be neat and well pressed and should fit well. Men should be clean-shaven, and women should wear minimal makeup. It is important that you remember that this is an excellent opportunity to make a good first impression on all of the individuals who review your deposition.

Because depositions are so important, we will reiterate here that, in deposition, you must avoid signs of annoyance or hostility, be forthcoming, and answer every question as well and concisely as possible. If you don't understand a question ask that it be repeated or rephrased until you do. Do not guess, do not try to outsmart the plaintiff's attorney, do not give vague answers or make unsolicited comments. Any of these can be trouble. Respond only to the specific questions asked; do not digress. No matter how experienced you might be as a physician, an expert witness or as a defendant, treat every deposition as a serious business interaction. Remember that plaintiff's attorneys are looking for inconsistencies in testimony, so the absolute truth is the best protection that one can afford him- or herself.

A key point to remember, if a case comes to trial, is that a jury is the "finder of fact." They determine what is true and thus determine the verdict in the case. You want the jury to like you. We repeat, you want the jury to like you! Be calm, professional in demeanor and forthcoming with your answers. It is important that you speak clearly and directly to them. In general, juries appreciate honesty, courtesy, professionalism and composure. We are aware of cases in which physicians, with the weight of the medical evidence on their side, have sabotaged their defense by being surly, arrogant, interrupting the plaintiff's attorney repeatedly, and making unwarranted remarks. Their resentment and indignation made them seem uncaring and mean spirited. Their hostile behavior made them unlikeable to the jury. Physicians repeatedly complain that lay juries are not qualified to sit in medical trials but, like it or not, it is the law. Despite that concern our experience is that the vast majority of lay medical malpractice case juries produce reasonable verdicts based on the facts of the case and how well the case was argued and presented by the litigators.

Juries are generally made up of middle-class individuals of modest to moderate means. They do not appreciate ostentatious exhibitions of wealth, arrogance, rudeness, or disregard; physicians that ignore the sensitivities of the average man or woman in medical practice or in the court room places themselves in peril.

Demeanor: the Projection of Confidence and Truthfulness

The most important things for a physician to project in a deposition are an air of professionalism and a high level of confidence and comfort. If the deponent can, with conviction, declare to the examiner and the camera that he has done nothing wrong, he has gone a long way in winning the battle of competing witnesses. The ability to project sincerity, confidence, and innocence are pivotal in disarming a plaintiff's case. The convincing defendant projects an aura of confidence that allows him to explain his conduct with self-assurance despite the arguments and tactics of the plaintiff's counsel.

The personal appearance of a physician at deposition or trial is of significant importance. At a deposition there are usually two lawyers, the deponent, and a legal transcriptionist; sometimes there is just a videographer; occasionally a transcriptionist and videographer. Some plaintiff's attorneys use a videographer to pressure a deponent. If a deponent physician appears stressed in deposition, the video may be introduced at trial. A calm smile and looking directly into the camera is very reassuring to observers.

Negative Feelings Produce Negative Responses from Observers

Many defendants are angry, hurt, and embarrassed by a medical malpractice claim. If you, as a defendant, are feeling defensive and angry, we urge you to get rid of those feelings before beginning any interactions with opposing counsel. Bring a negative attitude to a deposition and it will show through and hurt your credibility. A defensive deponent will find himself trying to justify actions rather than confidently recounting the events in question. Some defendants believe that, if they justify their actions in a deposition, they can convince the opposing counsel to drop the lawsuit. Unfortunately, they are wrong. The point for any deponent is to present himself as a confident and caring professional who did his best for the patient, despite a poor outcome.

When you are being examined, look the questioner in the eye. If being videotaped, look directly at the camera as much as you can. If you find yourself getting tired, upset, or angry, ask for a break. Don't let silly or repetitive questions bother you, because that is the norm in a deposition. Be prepared to hear some questions that don't make any sense at all. Don't answer unless you understand clearly. Remember this advice, "Never let opposing counsel see you sweat during a deposition".

What If There Clearly Has Been Malpractice?

When a poor therapeutic outcome in a patient's care occurs, we encourage a straightforward and sympathetic response from the involved physician(s) to the injured party and family. It has been our observation that injured parties are often grateful for the sympathy and empathy of their physician(s). They consider the physician(s) to be a friend(s). Important fact: injured parties are much less likely to sue friends than they are to sue someone from whom they feel distant or estranged. Failure to communicate with patients in many of these circumstances has led to unnecessary malpractice suits when the injured party and/or family has felt that a physician, or physicians, was being defensive or uncaring. A great sense of indignation and anger is raised when an individual feels ignored and abandoned, particularly by his or her health care professional. One may avoid malpractice claims by demonstrating caring behavior.

If there is a bad outcome due to obvious malpractice, and there is no way around accepting responsibility, we encourage defendants to be straightforward with their attorneys and make every effort to settle before the substantial expenses of litigation are incurred. If a plaintiff rejects settlement and it comes to the point where a deposition is to be taken, it is a good strategy for the defendant to humbly admit mistakes and *apologize* to the plaintiff. The act of contrition displays strength of character and a desire to do the right thing to anyone reading a deposition transcript or to the viewers of a videotape. Sincere remorse allows observers to feel *compassion and respect* for the defendant. A sincere apology can also open the door for the defendant to explain the extent of his responsibility and to describe the circumstances leading up to the plaintiff's misfortune. It may even give the defendant the opportunity to limit his culpability by not having to accept the entire responsibility for the unfortunate event. This can be a very good damage control strategy in a legal proceeding that would clearly go against the defendant.

When malpractice is obvious but the defendant stubbornly refuses to admit error, juries have been known to penalize the unrepentant tortfeasor with verdict awards that exceed their insurance limits. It is important that the defendant, whether innocent or guilty of medical malpractice, in every instance tell the truth in a convincing and sincere manner.

Uncertainty about the Ultimate Issue

If, in preparation for a deposition, you are not certain whether you breached the standard of care or not, we suggest that you carefully examine your actions as objectively as possible and without undue focus on the outcome. It is important to try and go back in time and determine the basis on which clinical decisions were made. We suggest that you consider writing out the entire scenario on paper, but *set this to paper only after asking the advice of counsel*. Work of this nature is not discoverable if specifically directed by counsel. If you do it without the advice of counsel, you might be creating evidence that could be used against you. Concentrate only on what you knew and actually did at the time. If, after analysis, you are satisfied that your actions were appropriate, you can confidently convey that feeling in a deposition or to a jury. If you are not wholly satisfied that you are not to blame, you must be willing to admit your errors while clearly explaining to your counsel what you did that you felt was right.

If this form of self-analysis leaves you uncomfortable regarding the propriety of some of your actions, talk about them with your attorney and explore legal and ethical ways of addressing your concerns. Under certain circumstances you may be able to truthfully testify, in good conscience, that the facts presented to you by the patient did not provide you with enough information to make an appropriate diagnosis or that the patient's actual diagnosis did not seem to be a plausible option at the time of presentation. To do this effectively you must show supporting data from concurring, generally accepted, medical sources.

Explanations, not Excuses

If a defendant physician's diagnostic and therapeutic plan has followed a recognized school of medical thought and his or her clinical decisions were based on accepted medical training and clinical experience, he or she is on solid ground for explaining his or her actions. Professional judgment does not have to be perfect, but it needs to reflect reasonable and prudent behavior. A defendant must demonstrate that diagnostic and therapeutic efforts were predicated on the information and conditions that were present at the time of the alleged malpractice.

We advise against making excuses in giving testimony. Juries do not take kindly to excuses of convenience, such as inadequate schedule time to see patients. Juries tend to believe that physicians have a specific duty to the patient before him or her and the failure to give that patient adequate care is inexcusable. Trying to place responsibility on others in a lawsuit also has its perils. For example, although you may rely heavily on nursing staff in practice, trying to shuffle care responsibility onto a nurse will hurt your defense unless it's obvious, in the record, that there was a clear and egregious nursing error. It serves no purpose to create an angry witness against you by antagonizing a co-worker unless there is clear evidence of the negligence of that associate.

One on One with the Other Side

Anyone who is deposed must accept the task of testifying as an opportunity to completely and honestly answer questions. Remember that the objective of opposing counsel is to discredit your testimony and eventually get into your bank account. The duty of plaintiff's counsel is to make every legal effort to put as much of your money as possible into his client's and his own pockets. Despite this knowledge, you must be courteous and professional in your behavior to opposing counsel whether you are being treated politely or harshly. Professional demeanor goes a long way in convincing others of your competence and honesty even in the face of adversity.

It is important for you to be aware that there are ways for you to defend yourself at a deposition. If you feel that a question is inappropriate or unfair, ask that it be repeated or rephrased. If there is any doubt whether a question is appropriate, your attorney will come to your aid by asking for clarification. You do not have to tolerate being demeaned or insulted by opposing counsel. If opposing counsel is overbearing or rude, ask him cease or ask the judge to intervene. Your counsel will also participate in protecting you should there be improper behavior by opposing counsel.

There are always questions posed that are not understood, so ask the attorney to rephrase them. If upon clarification you know the answer, give it truthfully, but do not guess or become involved in speculation. It is essential that you answer only the question asked and that you do not digress, because this can lead to additional questions that you may not want to answer. If it is clear that the plaintiff's lawyer doesn't understand the subject matter in question, it is not your duty to be his teacher. If you feel that you must explain an answer in detail, make sure that your explanation is well thought out and clearly presented. Don't be defensive, and do not, under any circumstances, loose your cool. Stay focused on the questions, not the questioner.

Do not go beyond your area of expertise in answering questions, because that can lead to questions that may adversely reflect on your competence, education and training. Some defendants make the error of trying to embellish credentials and experience in order to justify actions. That is a big mistake. It is better to focus on your established level of competence and skill rather than to suggest unverifiable credentials.

The majority of questions posed to a defendant usually focus on the differential diagnosis of the case in question. This will be particularly true if a part of the differential diagnosis was not carefully pursued in the work up and pursuit of the omitted portion would have been beneficial to the patient. That happens, not uncommonly, in complex medical and/or surgical case presentations. The problem can be minimized as a legal issue if, each time that you write a differential diagnosis, you demonstrate that the patient's work up is predicated on clinical impressions based on the patient's history, physical, and laboratory results. It is an excellent practice to note, next to each of the differential diagnoses, whether that particular option is likely or unlikely to be the definitive diagnosis. It is also wise to note the reasons for the prioritization. If a problem should arise in relation to the patient's care, someone may question your analysis but if in the notations you have demonstrated reasonable and prudent behavior in the assessment of the patient's problem, it is unlikely that you will be sued. Remember, you don't have to be perfect in your care, but you must demonstrate reasonable and prudent behavior, based on your education, training, and experience.

Deposition Preparation Advice

There are a number of books on the subject of how to prepare for depositions, but most of them are a waste of time. The best tip to keep in mind is that the best defense in a deposition is a good offense. If you are personally satisfied with the care provided the plaintiff, you can go on the offensive because you have nothing to hide.

Depositions—Preparation, Getting Ready for the Big Day

Depositions require a good deal of preparation before testifying. Here we touch on areas with which a deponent should be familiar. We will focus our attention on:

- Protected areas
- The patient's chart.
- Independent memory
- Habit and custom
- Physical evidence, such as laboratory studies, x-rays, etc.
- Common practices
- Articles and treatises
- Guidance on how to answer the tough questions.

Protected Areas—What Is Off Limits in a Deposition

It is worth repeating that every practicing physician should have an experienced trial lawyer with medical malpractice experience on retainer. That attorney should be the first person contacted when there is concern about a clinical matter with medicolegal implications. Concern may be based on an attorney's request for a copy of a patient's chart, a notice of investigation of a potential claim or a summons stating that a suit is being filed. In any of these circumstances the lawyer should be the first person contacted for guidance. Remember that all conversations with a personal attorney are privileged, confidential communications not subject to discovery by plaintiff's counsel or subject to discovery in deposition. A potential defendant can freely discuss his thoughts, feelings, and concerns with his lawyer regarding the matters in question without worrying that an opposing lawyer will find out about them. This is one of the best protections a defendant has in an adversarial proceeding. One can also do things related to a case in question upon "advice of counsel" without concern for discovery. On the other hand, discussions with one's own staff or other doctors are not privileged and are subject to discovery.

For example, suppose that you receive a summons or a letter implying a legal action regarding a patient on whom you have performed a minor procedure with reasonable but not perfect results. If, in anger and frustration, you vent your feelings about the matter to your staff and then discuss this with your partners or associates, all of those statements are discoverable. Your staff and other physicians can be deposed and asked about those statements. If, instead, you remain calm and realize that this is another cost of doing business and not the end of the world, you will be much better off. What you must do is to immediately call your lawyer to discuss the matter. That interaction is protected and so are the advice and the legal instructions given to you by your attorney in preparation for your defense.

As noted, all oral communications with counsel are shielded from discovery, as are written communications such as letters and memos produced by you at the request of counsel. On the other hand, memos or letters produced by you without the prior direction of counsel are not protected. Seek the advice of counsel before you write anything pertaining to the case at issue. If you independently write notes related to the case and place them in the patient's chart without your counsel's direction regarding those writings, plaintiff's lawyer can inquire about such notes and your counsel cannot have them excluded. Other items produced at the suggestion of counsel are likewise protected. These include time lines of events, typed transcripts of office notes, journal articles, and excerpts from textbooks, hospital and office records, and written recollection of events.

The Patients Chart—How the Medical Record Is Used

The notations that you or your staff make in a patient's medical record are generally accepted as gospel in a medical malpractice case. The reason for that is the legal presumption that patients divulge truth when seeking medical care and that the caregiver accurately records the information, test results, and other pertinent findings. This presumption allows medical expert witnesses to base their standard of care opinions on the medical record as it existed at the time it was made. Here we emphasize two important principles juries tend to believe:

- If it is written in the chart, it occurred as written.
- If it isn't written, it didn't occur.

Therefore, care and caution must be observed in all chart documentation. Avoid non-medical opinions and digressions.

It is impractical to record every detail of every examination and each verbal exchange, but it is very important to note all of the pertinent history. All of the history and the physical examination, along with the specific positives or negatives important to diagnosis and treatment, should be recorded. Brief notations related to pertinent positives and negatives will suffice but must be included in the physical assessment notes. It is a good practice to record the notes while the patient is with you. It is also a good practice to incorporate into your office record useful information received from other caregivers. If it is your custom and habit to have a nurse or another assistant record the patient's history, you should review it with the patient and, if you concur with the notations, you should note in your chart that you "concur with the history above." This confirms that you looked at and agreed with the history. If you feel the need to add to it or to correct it, make a note such as "history as above but patient states that fever started two days ago" and initial and date your addition If it is your clinical custom and habit to chart only positives, it may be assumed that unaddressed items are normal, negative, or not queried. On the other hand, it is better not to have a jury develop doubts as to what was and was not done in a patient's evaluation.

Accurate and Complete Medical Records

It is important to be careful in producing and recording medical records for many reasons. The main reason is that the information contained in a medical record belongs to the patient. The patient has the right to have an accurate record should he or she seek other medical care. If a medical record is illegible, the patient/plaintiff has the legal right to ask the physician/defendant for a complete and legible copy of the record.

The following will help to clarify the importance of accurate charting. In a recent malpractice case a urologist was charged with failure to appropriately follow a patient who had undergone prostate surgery. On a postoperative visit, the patient testified that he complained to the nurse of testicular swelling and pain. The doctor recorded no history and his only notation was "doing o.k." At an arbitration hearing the doctor tried to explain to the arbitrators that the note meant that everything was normal with the patient at the visit in question. To his regret, the statement was not accepted by the arbitration panel, which felt that the doctor had clearly disregarded the patient's history with subsequent injury to the patient.

Informed Consent Notations

An important element in every medical encounter is the issue of "informed consent." The law stipulates that a competent patient has control over his or body and the right to make a fully informed decision about any procedure that is to be undertaken on his or her person. The medical record must clearly reflect the fact that the patient has been appropriately informed of the risks, benefits, and alternatives, particularly to a proposed procedure. We recommend that each physician obtain informed consent on any procedure that he or she is to perform and clearly document the discussion. We advise against relying on ancillary personnel to obtain this consent. It is also recommended that a physician not indicate that an informed consent was obtained from a patient by noting it only in a surgical note. This can be damaging to the physician if it is the first appearance in the medical record and a bad result ensues.

When detailing the risks of a procedure to a patient, it is not necessary to list all of the risks. It is considered sufficient to explain the material (significant) risks of a procedure and ask if the patient understands those risks and wishes to proceed. If you have proceeded appropriately and obtained the consent of a well-informed patient, you should document that the "risks and benefits of the procedure as well as the alternatives were discussed with the patient." Note that the patient's concerns were addressed and that the patient understands the risks and wishes to proceed. This type of notation will avoid most claims of lack of informed consent.

Dictated Charts

Many physicians dictate their charts. If you do, we recommend that you carefully review the transcribed dictation and date and initial the chart if you agree with the content. If there are mistakes, write in your corrections on the chart, date and initial the changes. *Caution*: Do not make any corrections or other changes on a patient's chart after you learn that a legal claim has been raised. This is considered tampering with the record and can have serious legal consequences. One of the authors had a federal judge advise him, during a settlement conference, that he would allow the plaintiff to seek punitive damages against a physician client if the plaintiff could prove that the record had been modified to fit the doctor's statement of events.

If there is a delay of greater than 24 hours in transcription availability, it is wise to make temporary notations on the chart in lieu of the awaited encounter notes. The written note can be used by another health care provider if you are not immediately available or in case of an emergency. Problem lists, medication sheets, and an area for ordered labs in the chart provide others with a sense of your impressions and lines of investigation and treatment in the care of a patient.

Alterations to the Record

It is of utmost importance to again emphasize that the medical record must never be altered without using these appropriate procedures: initialing and dating any and all corrections and additions. No changes must ever be made after an attorney has requested records, because juries tend to be suspicious of alterations which may be self-serving and may thus impose punitive damages on the defendant.

In the era of electronic medical records, a new system for making corrections will have to be devised for each system utilized and by the institutions that utilize them. Office systems will likewise require correction/addition protocol procedures. In essence, the requirement of dating and initialing any change(s) in the medical record prevails no matter the method of recording data. It is all done to protect the well-being of the patient and to establish the care and prudence of the care giver.

Punitive Damages

Punitive damages are also called *exemplary damages*, because they are meant to set an example for others. They can be devastating because they are not covered by insurance and cannot be extinguished through bankruptcy. In a case of which we are aware, a physician went back to a hospital record and made changes above his original notes. He neither dated nor initialed the changes. His testimony was that the changes had been made immediately following the original writing of the notation. His claim was based on a photocopy of the chart. The claim fell on deaf ears when the original record was produced and revealed that the two notes were made in different colored inks. The result was a very large judgment against him and his hospital employer. If he had simply written the addendum, dated and initialed the changes, a different result would probably have occurred. The rule is very simple: charting must be done accurately. If corrections are made, do not change or alter the record. Write or type in the corrections somewhere on the chart or put a notation such as "see below" and then note the correction with the date and the initials of the person making the correction. It is also a good practice to note the time. All transcribed charts should be available as soon as possible and notes should be made on the chart in case interim care is needed.

Review All Pertinent Medical Records Prior to Deposition

When preparing for a deposition, thoroughly review the medical record and make sure that you can read and understand all the items included. Also, review hospital records that contain notes made by you but that are not in your possession or to which you do not have access. If there are problems in gaining access, because of institutional restrictions, they can be obtained by your counsel. The plaintiff usually provides authorization for access to the records.

There are few things more embarrassing to a physician than to admit that he cannot read his or her own handwriting, especially during a video deposition. That will almost guarantee that the video will be shown at trial and that a copy of the chart notes will be projected in the court room. Make sure that you can state what each notation in a chart says and what it means. You can count on the fact that you will be asked about each number, letter, and abbreviation on the chart. You will not be adequately prepared for deposition until you know the chart backward and forward and can read every word. If, after an examination, there is a word that you can't read but the meaning in context is obvious, admit the problem with the word and convey its clear meaning in other words.

If your records are handwritten, your counsel will probably request that you dictate each line of your record exactly as it is written, with annotations to explain specifically what the record means. This will help counsel understand your record and will aid in having an expert review the case for you. The note might look like this:

Abd.snb—chst, lgs,hrt-n-eent-n-t-100 hr/78

The transcribed note might look like this:

Abdomen soft, nontender; normal bowel sounds; chest, lungs, heart—normal; eyes, ears, nose, throat—normal; temperature 100; heart rate 78

This process also aids you in answering questions about the chart.

Documentation and Memory in the Legal Process

It is extremely rare for nurses, other office staff members, and physicians to recall the specifics of a patient's office visits. Because of this, it is acceptable for a physician to testify that he has no independent recollection of a specific visit. The doctor can testify to what is recalled from a particular visit, but most testimony is based on recollections derived from chart notes. There are three forms of memory that are legally recognized. These is actual memory, memory recorded, and memory refreshed. Actual memory is what is specifically remembered. Recorded memory is based on office notes and/or hospital records. Refreshed memory is memory that is refreshed by a document or writing that restores recollection of the event in question. In malpractice cases, recorded memory is most commonly used. Physicians are allowed to rely on their records during testimony because they deal with a wide variety of problems and many people.

Habit and Custom—What Is It and How Is It Used

All of us perform routine tasks on a daily basis without specific recollection of the particulars. If, for instance, you drive the same route to work daily, you probably won't recall the specifics of today's drive tomorrow, much less in a week. If asked, you would testify that you were on that road, if the day in question was a workday. The same is true in medical practice. If you routinely and habitually discuss with a patient the specific risks, benefits, and alternatives of a given procedure, you can comfortably testify that, based on your notations, that those issues were discussed. The same applies to a notation in the chart such as "history as above." This is an effective tool in a deposition or trial and is recognized by courts as a valid assertion of fact. The important thing is to establish that the activity is customary and habitual to your practice.

The patient's medical record may contain shorthand notations that can be explained under the category of customary and habitual practice. The notations are used to verify the assertion of custom and habit in patient care. For example, an abdominal exam may have revealed a soft, non-tender abdomen with normal bowel sounds. The chart may read "ab nbs". The notation may be meaningless to a layman but to you and other examiners it indicates that you examined the abdomen and noted your findings. Your testimony is bolstered when you testify from the record what you did and what you found. That testimony is based on habit and custom. We do recommend that if you use abbreviations in your charts, you be consistent and use only the ones found in one of the approved medical abbreviation dictionaries. It is important that other health care providers be able to interpret the notations should you not be available at a time the patient requires care.

Physical Tests—Uses and Dangers

With today's ever-expanding medical technology it has become standard practice to order multiple, complex, and expensive tests for patients. The necessity of much of that testing can be argued ad infinitum. Today's malpractice reality is such that, if certain tests are available to pursue a diagnosis being considered, they should be used or at least considered and so noted. If some of the tests are not ordered you may be in trouble if your diagnosis is wrong or if you have not ruled out a relevant illness. Misdiagnosis or failure to rule out a *life-threatening* diagnosis forms the basis of many lawsuits. For example, a cardiologist was sued for failure to order a CT scan on a patient who died from a thoracic aortic dissection hours after his discharge from an emergency department. The visit was initiated by abdominal discomfort. Neither the patient nor his wife informed the physician of a family history of heart and other vascular problems during the emergency department visit, history and physical examination. The patient's ECG and other tests were interpreted as normal; the patient's abdominal complaints resolved in the emergency department subsequent to administration of a GI cocktail. Despite the ECG and other tests used to rule out cardiac disease, the plaintiff's attorney argued that a CT scan of the chest would have revealed the lethal problem. Although the cardiologist was successfully defended at trial, the feeling of many physicians that one cannot do enough testing is perpetuated. It is not necessary to document reasons for not ordering every possibly relevant test in any given case. We do urge prudence and thoroughness in record keeping, reflected in the production of well-thought out notes in each patient's record. If a patient refuses a test helpful in making a diagnosis, reflect that in your notes. If you feel that a test is critical but the patient refuses to comply, request that he or she sign a waiver stating the reason for the refusal. If the patient declines to sign a waiver, be certain that you note that in the record. If there is no emergency, send a letter to the patient's last known address describing the reasons for the test or procedure as soon as possible. This establishes evidence regarding your effort to help the patient to make an appropriate medical decision. Place a copy of the letter in the chart.

When laboratory tests are ordered, be certain that the results are reviewed, dated, and initialed by an authorized member of the staff or by the attending physician before being placed in the patient's chart. If there are abnormal tests, record the fact that the patient was notified (date, time, and initials of the caller). It is a good practice to ask patients to call your office about all test results, but, when a test is abnormal, it is imperative that you or your staff inform the patient promptly in order to initiate the appropriate follow up. There is no desire to frighten patients, but prompt attention and follow up on abnormal results gives patients confidence in your concern for their well-being.

When blood, x-rays, ECGs or other tests are sent to a specialist or laboratory, you are depending on the expertise of the individual or laboratory for an accurate assessment of the materials sent. In law you have the right to rely on the report of the expert that interpreted the tests. When reports are received, note in the chart the date and time reviewed and any pertinent thoughts. Normal reports are particularly important, as they are considered to be a "pertinent negative" in a work-up.

In case of emergency or serious acute illness when immediate results are required, it is unacceptable practice to order out-of-the-office testing. Under these circumstances it is imperative to send the patient to a hospital laboratory or to an emergency unit and to follow up on the laboratory results as soon as they are available. As an example, a physician was sued because of ordering laboratory tests that would not be reported until the following day. The physician correctly suspected a bacterial infection in a patient with a three-day history of high fever, nausea, vomiting, and diarrhea. Blood for culture and sensitivity was drawn and sent to a local laboratory for overnight processing. It was clear that the physician had to know that the results would not be available until the next morning. Unfortunately, by the time the results were available the patient was in critical condition and died of an overwhelming sepsis on the way to a hospital. The claim against the physician was predicated on the severity of the patient's illness, inadequate treatment due to failure to confirm his suspicions by immediate testing and the failure to hospitalize the patient despite the suspicion of a grave illness.

Rural Practice Standard Exceptions

Because there are now accepted national standards for medical care, common or local practice standards are of little value in most malpractice cases. Occasionally, the issue of local standards does pop up. This arises in cases in which medical care and/or hospitalization occurred in a rural area without access to medical experts or services in each of the specialty fields applicable to the case. In rural practice areas questions may arise regarding the level of care provided and what is expected of other rural care providers under the same or similar circumstances. For example, it is generally agreed that, even in a city, it can take from 30 to 60 minutes to assemble and prepare an emergency surgical team for action. The circumstances of location, resources and medical care options can alter the level of care accessibility. In rural areas the standard of care may differ somewhat from that of a city and, to some extent, the legal concept of a local standard may apply. Despite that exception, practicing medicine in a rural area today requires that reasonable logistical plans to deal with the very ill be in place. When circumstances preclude the implementation of those plans but conscientious effort is made to provide the best available care on site, allowances are made. The law is neither entirely blind nor heartless. When a physician follows the standards and common practices of others in his or her specialty in similar localities and similar circumstances, there is generally little difficulty in convincing a jury of the competence of the physician involved.

Articles and Treatises—How to Prevent Damage

In deposition it is likely that the defendant physician will be asked to name the journals that he or she regularly reads. The purpose of this line of questioning is to allow the plaintiff's attorney and the plaintiff's expert witnesses to review those journals to see if they contain articles that address the issues in the lawsuit. If you are the defendant, you may be asked at trial if you are familiar with a specific article in one of those journals, whether you agree that the article is authoritative and whether you agree with certain statements contained in the article. *This is very important to know;* if you agree that the article in question is authoritative, you may put yourself into a corner unless you did everything exactly as the author suggested. On the other hand, you may truthfully state that the article in question is the author's view and that you may or may not agree with the conclusions. If you state that the article is not authoritative that may end the inquiry in some jurisdictions, but be ready to explain why. The authoritativeness of source materials is a subject to be seriously discussed with defense counsel prior to deposition. If asked to agree or disagree with the authoritativeness of particular articles, make sure to review and understand them prior to answering at deposition. If you have not studied the materials in question, do not answer the question.

The same rules apply to journal articles on the subject in question. You can agree that portions are authoritative while others are not. Keep in mind that books and even journal articles may be outdated by the time they are printed. It is also true that the circumstances under which an author works may be totally different from those faced by you at the time of the alleged malpractice. If asked about a book on your shelf, it is well to admit that it is a reference tool used on occasion to help in your practice, but it is reasonable to testify that, based on your education, training, and experience, you do not limit yourself to treating patients based on the information contained in a single text.

Some books on medical malpractice provide readers with a list of questions to prepare them for deposition or trial. We are not going to list a number of tough questions that have caused consternation to physicians. We feel that the variety of questions and the way in which they are asked vary so much that putting together a top 40 list is inane. The way to be thoroughly prepared for a deposition or trial is to work diligently with your attorney and review the medical records carefully. If after thorough study you can honestly answer "no" to the question "Did you do anything wrong," you have little to fear. Armed with knowledge and firm in your conviction that you did nothing wrong, you can answer any question posed with conviction and comfort. Beyond that sense of confidence, never forget that it is important that you are seen as professional, competent, and caring.

In the course of a deposition and/or trial testimony, you will be asked whether you did or did not consider some element in the patient's assessment to be important. You must be prepared to answer clearly and with conviction. For example, an obstetrician may be asked why he or she did not consider a portion of a fetal monitor strip to be abnormal. It is important to be clear and specific in explaining in order to communicate to the jury why a certain course of care was chosen over another. The hard questions are always "why" and "why not" inquiries.

There are a number of books on the market on how to prepare for depositions. One of the authors had such a book that a defendant physician asked to read prior to his deposition.

Although the physician was discouraged from reading the book, he insisted. After the deposition was scheduled, a follow-up meeting was scheduled with the defendant to be held the day prior to the deposition in order to complete preparations for testifying. In the interim, the physician had read the book and developed what we call "paralysis of analysis." He called prior to the scheduled deposition and stated that he needed more time to prepare because of what he had read. The deposition was rescheduled but, in a couple weeks, the doctor called again saying that he felt that he would never be ready. He was fighting a war within himself, and he could not prepare his mind to be straightforward and truthful in his testimony. He wanted a formula that guaranteed success. He wanted to outwit the plaintiff's attorney rather than cooperate and testify truthfully, a very dangerous venture. He had developed the mindset that he wasn't going to give an inch in his testimony; that attitude pointed to the disaster that the deposition became. In his effort to "concede nothing to the plaintiff's lawyer," as the book had advised, he testified during the deposition that a patient with a blood pressure of 0 over 0 was not necessarily in shock. No need to divulge the outcome of the legal process here, as you have already sorted that out and the book disappeared, never to be seen again. The fact is that the law is not a game to be played, no matter the source of knowledge. There is no legal strategy that trumps honesty, sincerity, and truth.

Production of Documents

As mentioned above, during discovery, documents are exchanged by the attorneys when a request is sent by one attorney to the other listing certain documents and/or records that the other side would like to review. In a malpractice case the documents most commonly requested by plaintiff's counsel are the patient's complete file, billing records, photographs (if any), the defendant's C.V., any correspondence related to the case, and the defendant's liability insurance policy. This process is handled by the attorneys, so there is no need to go into detail. Most states have adopted rules that require the opposing sides to locate and copy documents that may be relevant to the claim being made.

Request for Admissions

Requests for admissions is a legal maneuver, the purpose of which is to have the opposing side admit the truth of relevant matters and avoid having to prove those matters at trial. In general, the request is limited to matters that are material (i.e., relevant to the case) but not privileged. You may be asked, for example, to admit that you ordered a specific test for the patient on a certain day. Your answer is to admit or deny the truth of the allegation or state why you can neither admit nor deny the truth. How you respond to these questions is best left to counsel on a case-by-case basis. Suffice it to say that an affirmative response to a request for admissions will be used at trial if it helps to prove the plaintiff's case. Be sure to ask your attorney why each request is being admitted or denied and the probable consequences of the submitted answers to the case.

Physical Examinations

Most courts allow defense attorneys to arrange for an independent medical examination of a plaintiff. This is to help determine whether or not the plaintiff's current medical condition and care is related to the negligence claim against the defendant. Because the injuries alleged in malpractice cases are generally known to the defense, independent examinations are not commonly performed. Defense attorneys don't request independent medical examinations because that may provide the plaintiff with the opportunity to have the claim against the defendant reiterated by another physician, i.e., the physician hired by the defense. If the independent examiner is called as a witness at trial, the patient's history will be used by the plaintiff's counsel to have the defense witness describe the plaintiff's complaint to the jury. Because most plaintiffs seek follow-up care from other physicians, it is often easier and safer to depose the patient to ascertain his perception of his current medical condition and how his current status was negatively affected by the defendant's care. Whether or not to request an independent medical examination is a complicated question that you need to discuss with counsel.

Alternative Dispute Resolution

Alternative dispute resolution involves settlement of cases by legal means other than trial. These alternative methods come into play when a complaint has been filed, but non-judicial methods of case resolution are chosen in an effort to avoid a trial and the costs of litigation. These methods include court-ordered settlement conferences, arbitration (binding and non-binding), and mediation. Each of these methods will be discussed separately. Claims settled prior to a lawsuit being filed will not be discussed.

Settlement Conferences

In some local and state jurisdictions and in the federal courts, a trial judge may order a settlement conference. The plaintiff and counsel, the defendant and counsel, and, on occasion, a representative of the defendant's insurance carrier are invited to meet with the judge to discuss a possible resolution. This type of conference is informal; no records are kept. In this setting the trial judge may initially meet with the counsel for each side to see what progress can be made toward resolution. There is often some arm twisting by the judge in these conferences, with a lot of emphasis on the expense and the risk of litigation to both sides. These sessions can be effective if the defendant is willing to settle and the plaintiff is reasonable in his demands. At these conferences legal positions are weighed by both parties, and each must decide on the strength of his or her case and chances of success at trial. If either side is recalcitrant, the case will not settle. Even if there is no settlement, these sessions are frequently valuable, because the parties can agree to certain stipulations of fact and may resolve certain trial issues and thus limit the scope and the length of a trial. As in every other type of legal proceeding, it is important for the physician to be fully aware, prior to the time of the meeting, of the nature of the settlement conference, of what may be accomplished in conference, and of what his or her other options are.

Arbitration

Arbitration is a formal hearing of the facts in a case before an impartial individual or a panel, usually made up of three persons, sworn to try the case fairly and impartially and render an award to the side that presents the more compelling case. Usually, there is agreement between counsel for the parties to use the written reports of some experts that they have hired rather than having all of the possible witnesses testify. In most arbitration, the plaintiff, the defendants, and the expert witnesses, who establish the standard of care, do testify. There is also agreement to use medical records without the need for subpoenas. The purpose of arbitration is to shorten the legal process and avoid a trial while still presenting all relevant and material evidence. The manner and method of presenting evidence in arbitration is worked out by the attorneys, and, in general, a fair and accurate presentation of the facts occurs.

Arbitration is binding only when the parties agree to be bound by the award prior to the hearing. If there is agreement to binding arbitration, the agreement is usually filed with the court. After the hearing the prevailing party will file the arbitration award and ask for a court order confirming the award. In the case of binding arbitration there is no appeal from the arbitration decision, and the case ends with the award.

Arbitration is non-binding when either party has a right to appeal the award to a trial court and proceed to a jury trial. Court-ordered arbitration is usually non-binding but requires that the litigants appear and present their respective sides of the question. Some jurisdictions have court rules that allow the non-binding arbitration award (the arbitrator's decision) to be presented to a jury should a lawsuit be initiated. In order for the arbitration award to be presented to a jury, certain requirements must be met, such as the failure to present a defense to the plaintiff's charges at the arbitration hearing.

If an arbitration panel is offered by a court as a means of dispute resolution, we recommend that the offer be declined because there is an inherent problem of bias in the panel selection process. Panels are established by the plaintiff's attorney and the defense attorney each selecting one member to serve on the panel. It is then up to the two selected arbitrators to identify a mutually acceptable third arbitrator. The selection process clearly puts the panel's decision in the hands of the third arbitrator because the two initially chosen panelists are usually biased toward the side that chose them. As this is frequently the case, we encourage the use of a single, well-respected, arbitrator who can be fair and unlikely to render an extravagant award to the plaintiff if that side should prevail. At the end of the arbitration process, there will be a written decision based only on the facts presented and reflecting the thought processes of the arbitrator. This is put forth to accomplish resolution of the dispute.

Mediation

Meditation is another non-judicial method of dispute resolution that is gaining favor in malpractice cases. It is usually a court-ordered process and is non-binding. In this procedure the court selects the individual who will act as the mediator. The mediator is not required to have any experience in malpractice litigation to be effective. He has only to be impartial, because the essence of mediation is finding a settlement that both parties can accept. Once mediation has been ordered and the mediator has been selected, the only requirement, other than a time and place for a meeting, is that the parties and their representatives be present. In mediation there is agreement by the parties that everything said during the sessions is confidential and that nothing said by either side can later be used at trial. This affords the opportunity for the parties to hear and understand the position of the other side. In addition to hearing the other side's positions and interests, each side has the opportunity to assess how its own case will sound to a jury should it become necessary to go to trial. The sides can determine whether their cases are weak or strong and whether it is worth exposing themselves to a directed resolution imposed upon them by a court.

Mediation begins with the mediator laying out the ground rules. These rules are based on the premise that the parties are interested in reaching settlement. The mediator will ask counsel for the plaintiff to present his case and to indicate what his side expects to be able to prove at trial. The mediator may question the plaintiff about the case, which is the main reason for confidentiality. After the mediator has an understanding of the claim against the physician, the physician's attorney is then asked to make the defense presentation. Again, the mediator may question the physician about certain aspects of the case. After a session with all parties present, the mediator meets separately with both sides to see if a settlement can be reached. The mediator does not take a direct part in the decision-making process but tries to help the parties focus on aspects of the case on which they can agree. If the sides are willing to make concessions, the process of settlement begins. An effective mediator meets individually and frequently with both parties during the process. The mediator conveys messages between the parties and suggests possible areas of mutual interest that can lead to settlement. After the process has been completed, the mediator will bring the parties together to ascertain whether the parties agree to a resolution. Subsequently, an announcement is made as to whether a settlement has or has not been reached. If a settlement is agreed upon, a memorandum is drafted and signed by the parties. The memo stipulates the particulars of the agreement and establishes legal grounds for its performance.

Preparation for Alternative Dispute Resolution

The determining factor in deciding whether to participate in alternative dispute resolution is an honest appraisal of the case against you. If you have failed on the motion to dismiss the case and you are headed for trial, you must realize that the case could be decided against you. If you and your attorney place the odds of winning at 50/50 or less, you must be serious in your effort to resolve the litigation. Do not let the decision be based on extraneous issues such as the National Practitioner Data Bank and the possible effect of a settlement on your standing in the medical community. It is easier to explain a $50,000 settlement in the face of a strong case than to explain a $1,000,000 verdict. You must also keep in mind that the press likes to report a big verdict against a prominent physician while settlements are rarely reported. You must also keep in mind that a settlement that requires that neither party disclose the terms of the settlement can be reached. In addition, the malpractice attorney appointed by the insurance company and your liability insurance representative have a role in determining what is to be reported. With these things in mind, most prudent attorneys will tell a client in jeopardy of losing a malpractice action that it is best to settle a bad case. We strongly stress careful preparation for any dispute resolution. In arbitration the objective is to win. Anything less is not acceptable. In mediation, while you want to impress the other side with your understanding of their position, you must also be prepared to emphasize the weakness of their case and the strength of yours. Prepare for arbitration as you would for trial and prepare for mediation as you would for a college debate.

Pre-Trial Conferences

A pre-trial conference is a formal meeting of the attorneys for the two sides to discuss the upcoming trial before the trial judge. At this conference the claim of the plaintiff, the defense to that claim, the testimony of witnesses to be called at trial, exhibits to be introduced, and the position of the parties on potential settlement are discussed. After the conference the attorneys will have a good idea as to the trial date. It is important that you consult with your counsel as soon as the pre-trial conference is completed so that you can begin to make scheduling plans for your office and personal activities.

In most jurisdictions, attorneys must file a pre-trial statement that sets forth his or her version of the facts; lists the trial issues to be decided by the jury; identifies the witnesses to be called, with a brief summary of their expected testimony; and identifies exhibits that the party plans to offer. If the trial judge so orders, other pertinent matters may be included in the pre-trial statement. The attorneys prepare their pre-trial statements with little input from their clients. If you are a defendant in a malpractice case, make certain that your attorney provides you with a draft copy of his proposed statement for your review and comment prior to its formal submission to the court. You have the right to see what is being filed on your behalf and to discuss it with your counsel. If you have concerns about the statement, address them to your counsel. Although the statement is a legal formality, you will want to make sure that you and defense counsel are of the same mind as to the position you will be taking at trial. You will want to receive a copy of the pre-trial statement that is actually filed to put it in your litigation file and a copy for your personal attorney.

Both sides must submit pre-trial statements to the court, so ask your counsel to mail a copy of the plaintiff's statement to you for review and comment. This will help you to understand what the plaintiff's side is claiming at trial and how it proposes to prove its case. Even though your counsel will understand the scope of the claim, you must make certain that you are clearly aware of all of the elements of the case to be presented before the trial begins. Make sure that a copy of every pre-trial statement is sent to your personal counsel as well.

In some jurisdictions, the trial judge requires that the plaintiff and defendant appear along with their legal counsel for the pre-trial conference. If this situation applies to your case, make sure that you meet with counsel to discuss the process and how you should handle yourself. At the pre-trial conference, you may receive a lot of pressure from the trial judge to settle the case, so be prepared to discuss your position in a matter-of-fact way with the judge. If you are firm in your belief that you did nothing wrong and can express that feeling to the judge, you will have no problem. Judges sometimes tell horror stories about other cases where "bad things happened to a doctor just like you." This is done to try to generate a settlement and avoid a trial. Listen intently but don't let the "war stories" affect your resolve. As stated above, settle a case if it is clear that the case against you is strong and your defense weak, but stay the course if you are in the right and your defense is strong. There is no virtue in defending a losing position to the end.

The Trial—Getting Ready for the Big Contest

Preparation

Scheduling

Planning is the linchpin of good trial preparation. The first thing you will want to know is the trial date and the expected length of the trial. If the court system in which the case will be heard has a trailing docket, a number of cases set for the same date, you will need to ask how likely it is that your case will go forward on the scheduled date. If you are uncertain as to whether the case will proceed or not, you may want to make contingency plans that will allow you to have a light appointment schedule for that week. Back-up appointments can be set up in the event that the case is continued, i.e., set to a later time. Changing trial dates, with at least one continuance, is the norm in many jurisdictions. Your attorney should be aware of the court's schedule; some courts routinely do not try cases on Fridays, and some courts are in session only part of the day. Once you are certain of the trial date and the usual court schedule, begin your final pre-trial preparations.

We suggest that you cancel all appointments for all of the days affected for a trial that is projected to last a week or less. This is expensive, but it will enable you to be rested and not distracted during the trial. If you have no alternative to seeing patients on those days, you may arrange to see patients in the mornings and evenings. If the trial is scheduled to last more than a week, try to schedule patients in the evenings or on weekends. Our best advice is to make every effort to completely free up the evening before you testify. You want to be well rested when you take the stand. You'll want to be calm and collected and free from work-related distractions; we want you to be the best witness that you can possibly be. You will be the most important witness for the defense.

Familiarity with the Record

Just as we suggested in the section on preparation for the deposition, the most important thing that you will want to do is to thoroughly review the patient's chart and familiarize yourself with every detail. Make certain that you understand the case thoroughly. During the process of preparation you, with your attorney's help, should produce a chronological time line of the events in question. You will want to have the sequence of events clearly in your mind. We recommend that you begin the review about two weeks prior to the trial. Make as many notes as you need, under the direction of your attorney. Plan to rely on the patient's medical record as the basis for your testimony at trial. Remember that the medical record and any other notes that you may need can be taken with you to the stand and can be used for reference during testimony. Remember also that the counsel for the other side has the right to review whatever you bring to the witness stand. It is best to have only the medical record and a copy of your discovery deposition with you.

Feel free to use the medical record as much as necessary. Do not be concerned that a jury might feel that you are uninformed. If you are familiar with the chart and can answer most questions from memory that will reinforce the jury's perception of your competence. It is a good practice to refer to the chart when plaintiff's counsel asks very specific questions. For example, you might answer a question about the date of the first visit by answering, "I believe that I first saw the patient on June 4, 2010, but, let me verify that from the chart." You can then look at the chart to confirm the date. You will be asked specific questions about the record, so be sure you are able to read and explain its contents. Opposing counsel frequently enlarges portions of records for projection and will ask questions from the enlargements. When that occurs you may refer to your copy of the chart or the enlargement for your answers. Use whichever makes you more comfortable. Although it is your attorney's responsibility to make sure that the enlargement is accurate, it is a good practice to compare the original and the enlargement to make sure that you are dealing with an accurate copy.

Preparing to Testify

Once you are completely familiar with the chart, you will want to concentrate on reviewing your discovery deposition. Remember that most questions from the plaintiff's counsel at trial will come from the medical record and the discovery deposition. For that reason, we suggest that you schedule plenty of quiet time to thoroughly review your discovery deposition. You will need to be very familiar with that document. Read it several times. The first review, in preparation for trial, should be to get a broad grasp of content. Make no effort to second guess your deposition answers. You don't have to like it, just read it. Don't make notes at that time. It is important to understand that we write differently than we speak, so don't be surprised if what you read in the deposition sounds a bit foreign to you.

Several days after reading the discovery deposition, get some paper, a pencil, and a highlighter and review the deposition a second time. This time look at the specific questions and answers. If, as you read, you are satisfied with your response move on to the next question. When you come to a question and answer that you feel is of special importance, highlight it for further study and preparation. After highlighting areas that you feel are important, go back and ask yourself if you are satisfied with the answers. Consider whether you wish you had elaborated further. If there are areas that you feel could be better explained, write your expanded comments either on the deposition text or on note paper with reference to the page and line numbers in the deposition. You should schedule time to go over these notes with your counsel prior to trial. If the answers were satisfactory don't try to become too fine in making a point. Your purpose is simply to refine your responses in harmony with your prior testimony. If you can say the same thing with more specificity or rearrange the wording to reflect more clearly your answer, you are on the right track. If you find an error in prior testimony, you can make a clarifications and/or correction to the prior testimony as long as you tell the truth. No human is perfect, and juries tend to understand if you explain that a previous answer wasn't accurate due to misunderstanding of a question or a failure to comprehend the whole picture at the time of deposition. On the other hand, juries do not like trial testimony that is clearly contradictory to prior sworn testimony. If there is any question, the plaintiff's attorney will have your deposition testimony read back to you. You don't want your trial testimony to vary significantly from your sworn deposition testimony.

The next thing in this process of self-evaluation is to assess your overall performance at the deposition. You need to be as objective as possible regarding your strengths and weaknesses. After having read, highlighted, and evaluated the testimony, you will have a feeling for those areas of testimony in which you were comfortable and those areas where you were not. Even if you feel comfortable with your overall deposition performance, take a second look. It is very difficult to be completely objective in self-evaluation, but we want you to judge just how you will be perceived by a jury. You want the jury to see you as professional, competent, thoughtful and caring. It is important not to be seen as arrogant, uncaring, flippant, or unprofessional. Consult with your attorney and ask for criticisms, suggestions, and coaching. This is all part of the preparation for trial. Your attorney is on your side and will be happy to help you to be as good a witness as possible.

Meeting with Personal Counsel

When you have completed your review of the deposition, you will discuss what you've done with counsel and determine how to address any concerns that you may have before trial. We advise you to follow counsel's advice but, you must be comfortable with it. If you are not at ease, discuss your concerns until you are. You will be testifying, not the lawyer, and it is your comfort that is most important. Problem questions likely to be asked by plaintiff's counsel should be asked and answered in practice sessions with counsel, but that process is best left to his or her judgment. Rehearsals are a way of providing comfort for the defendant and not a time for creating new evidence. The focus must be on telling the truth in a compelling and clear way to the jury.

When you and legal counsel are satisfied that you are ready, prepare an outline of your testimony. By this we mean outline the areas of your testimony that will be covered, on direct examination, by your attorney while you are on the stand. During your testimony your attorney should follow the outline so that you will feel confident as to where he is going. If you are on the same wavelength, your testimony will flow smoothly and that enhances credibility.

Once you and your counsel feel that you are prepared, our best advice to you is to try to relax, get plenty of rest, and make every effort to put the trial out of your mind. At this point, you will have done all that is within your control, and no amount of worry or second guessing is going to help. Avoid too much coffee, alcohol or sedating medications. We want a calm and confident witness on the stand.

How Do I Dress for Trial

As we've mentioned previously, the jury expects a professional appearance; don't disappoint them. The dress for female physicians may be a pantsuit, a business suit, or a dress. Skirts must extend below the knees. Makeup and accessories should be modest and add a taste of class. Male physicians have no options other than a modest, well-fitting, well-pressed dark suit when they take the stand. On days when not on the stand, a sport coat and slacks with an appropriate tie and shirt will pass muster but a suit is still preferable. Male physicians should avoid jewelry beyond a wedding ring, a class ring and a modest watch. For the female physician, simple earrings, a wedding band or similar ring, a simple watch or bracelet, and a modest necklace are appropriate. Shoes should be modest, shined and with heels of no more than two inches. Nails should be well manicured and hair should appear well combed and cared for. We advise physicians not to change their appearance significantly during trial and, if there was a video deposition, to try to keep their appearance pretty much the same as it was at that time.

How Do I Act

We cannot tell you why it is true—there are no controlled studies to substantiate what we are about to say—but our observations and experiences have convinced us that juries pick up on subtle fears, hostilities, and prejudices that are brought into the courtroom. Our advice is for you to relax and come to the courtroom with a feeling that you have nothing to hide or fear. "That's easy for you to say" (you may be thinking), but, from this point forward, many things are going to occur that are completely out of your control. You can only control your behavior and testimony. If you believe in yourself and your position, let all else go, and relax. There is no doubt that you can lose a case with a bad attitude, and it is equally true that you can help yourself by being personable and professional in demeanor. You probably won't prevail simply because you're a nice person, but it won't hurt your case to be so. Realize that your counsel is in charge at this point and that you have a supporting role, not the lead, to play in the trial. Concentrate on being a good witness, and forget everything else. Relax, take a deep breath, and walk into the courtroom.

Trial—the Tribulation

At this point we are ready to begin to lay out the scenarios of a trial. A trial is a real-life drama played out before a jury that, in theory, knows nothing about the case before it and knows none of the parties. The trial is presided over by a judge. The judge is the *hearer of law*, who decides what evidence the jury can hear and who instructs the jury as to the law that is applicable to the case. The jury is designated the *hearer of fact*. The evidence that a jury hears establishes the basis for its verdict. The evidence is provided by the accounts of witnesses and from exhibits and/or documents that the trial judge allows the jury to see. When the required number of jurors agrees, a verdict is reached and the trial is over.

Trials have requisite legal sequences that are followed in almost all jurisdictions. The legal events that make up a trial are presented below. After an introductory statement by the judge, the following events take place:

- Impaneling a jury.
- Voir dire.
- Opening statements by the counsels for the parties.
- Calling of witnesses and receiving of evidence.
- Closing arguments, also called summation.
- Jury instructions from the trial judge.
- Jury deliberations.
- Reading of the verdict.

Impaneling a Jury

Most state courts select potential jurors from the list of registered voters in the county in which the trial is to be held. Sometimes other records, such as driver's license registrations, are used. Jurors must reside in the county or district in which the trial will take place. Prospective jurors are assigned numbers that are drawn at random by the Clerk of Courts to determine which jurors may be called for jury duty during the term of court. The term of a court usually lasts from three weeks to two months. Each prospective juror is sent a questionnaire by the Clerk of Courts that requires him or her to identify him- or herself and give his or her occupation, level of education, marital status, age, prior jury experience, any lawsuit involvement, etc. These questionnaires are generally available to counsel for the parties from a day to a week prior to trial. These responses are invaluable in determining the general makeup of the panel. If juror questionnaires are used in your jurisdiction, it is imperative that you review them with counsel prior to trial so you can identify, in advance, any potential jurors whom you know or whose family members are familiar to you. It is important to avoid juror bias.

Jury selection is of great importance, so meet with your counsel prior to the jury's being seated and discuss the type of jurors that you would like to see impaneled. Go over the questions, with counsel, that the attorneys and judge are likely to ask prospective jurors. You may suggest question to your counsel that you think may be important to the selection of an unbiased jury panel. During questioning, look at each juror and ask, "Is this a juror who will be fair and impartial or is this a juror that causes concern." Make a note regarding your perceptions of each juror and later discuss those notes with counsel. You will never get the perfect jury but you want a fair and impartial panel that will consider all of the facts within the time frame and the circumstances in which they occurred.

Be observant during the process of jury selection but do not openly participate. Listen to all of the questions and responses but don't talk to counsel during the process unless absolutely necessary. If there are reasons for concern, speak with counsel after the questioning period is completed. Finally, remember that if a preemptory challenge is made due to a voir dire response, the responses of the next juror to be seated must be considered. If a juror is excused because of a particular response to a question, it is important to be aware that the following juror could be even more of a problem to your side.

Voir Dire

Prior to voir dire, the judge predicts the length of the trial so that prospective jurors unable to commit themselves for the anticipated length of the trial can be identified. Most judges will allow people who have substantial and verifiable hardship problems to be discharged.

The phrase comes from the French and translates as "truth telling." During this phase of the trial, the judge has the prospective jurors sworn to answer truthfully all questions posed to them. The questions deal with the ability to sit as fair and impartial jurors in the case at hand. After the prospective jurors are sworn, the trial judge, in state courts, will introduce the parties to the suit and their counsel and ask if jurors know the parties in litigation or the witnesses or have knowledge of the facts of trial. These questions are designed to prompt any juror who may know or be familiar with the case at hand to come forth. If a prospective juror comes forth at this point, he is usually disqualified because of likely biases.

After the judge has completed his or her inquiries related to seating a jury, counsel for the plaintiff followed by counsel for the defense are allowed to pose questions to the panel. This is a very important part of the trial, as it is the only time that counsel can actually speak with each juror and inquire as to their qualifications. Voir dire usually takes several hours.

There are two ways to exclude individuals from a particular jury. The first is a *challenge for cause* and the second is a right known as a *preemptory challenge*. The challenge for cause is used to prohibit certain citizens from sitting on a jury because of felony convictions or other legislative prohibitions. Challenge for cause of this type is rarely used. Challenge for cause can be exercised, by either party, when a juror claims that he or she cannot be fair, knows or is related to a party or a material witness, is currently a client of one of the lawyers, or is a patient of a defendant. These challenges are raised by counsel and are decided by the trial judge. Cause challenges are frequently discovered while reviewing the juror questionnaires prior to voir dire. They may also be the product of questions raised by the judge or counsel prior to seating the jury.

The peremptory challenge is the right of counsel for either side to excuse any juror for any reason without explanation. There are limits to that right. Lawyers are prohibited from trying to sanitize a jury, i.e., tip the balance of a jury to their favor by excluding qualified jurors. Each side generally has three peremptory challenges. After the panel has been questioned by the court and opposing counsel, the judge will ask each attorney whether any juror will be challenged. If a juror is challenged, he or she is excused and the next eligible juror is placed on the panel. The right starts with the plaintiff, followed by the defendants, back to the plaintiff, etc. until the challenges are exhausted. When completed, the panel is set.

Peremptory challenges are extremely important in jury selection, and the defendant should be involved in that process. For example, a defendant will want to excuse an otherwise qualified juror who is considering filing a malpractice suit or who has a history of a number of lawsuits. A nurse or other health care professional could be an asset or a liability, depending on the issues raised. The circumstances under which peremptory challenges are used are many and varied and require serious consideration.

Opening Statement

This is the opportunity for each side to explain to the jury its perception of what the case is about. In general, it is a recitation of what each side expects the evidence to prove at trial. It is not permissible to argue the case at this point. The opening statement is like the outline of a book or a road map designed to give the jury background information to understand what each side is claiming. Opening statements are crucial in civil cases. It is claimed by many experienced attorneys that more than half of all jurors make up their minds about a case on the basis of the opening statements. Attorneys try to combat this tendency by impressing on juries in voir dire that they must not make up their minds until they have heard all of the evidence and received the judge's instruction on the applicable law.

Although the opening statement is purely a lawyer's function, it is important that you discuss with counsel what he or she will say. Most attorneys memorize their opening statements so that they can present a smooth and compelling narrative. What is vital in an opening statement is the clarity of the presentation. Some lawyers are better than others in this phase of trial. The jurors are told in advance by the judge that what the lawyers say in the opening statement is not to be considered as evidence but only as background information to help the jury understand the nature of the controversy. Because clarity is important in the opening statement, you want to make sure that you and your attorney agree on the basic elements of the presentation.

During opening statements you will want to be attentive to what opposing counsel tells the jury about its case. Look attentive and do not make notes. It is your responsibility to appear confident and professional. Do not betray negative emotion to what you are hear. Make mental notes of opposing counsel's statements with which you don't agree or hear for the first time. These can then be addressed with your counsel during a trial recess.

As soon as the opening statements are finished, meet with your counsel to address any concerns. It is your attorney's job to help you deal with any concerns that you may have. His understanding of the process can help in allaying fears. All defendants are anxious, but if you are convinced that you have not been negligent, you will be able to handle the stresses of a trial. Alarm or fears can dampen your confidence, so discuss your concerns honestly with counsel. The worst thing you can do is to disregard disquieting remarks presented by the plaintiff's attorney in his opening statement without some discussion with your counsel. If a surprising statement is uttered in the opening you can be sure it will be brought up in cross examination before the jury. You don't want to be caught unprepared on the stand, so be sure that you and your counsel have prepared to deal with any relevant issue.

Evidence and Witnesses

A trial is the presentation of evidence as testimony of witnesses and through the use of exhibits such as a patient's chart, hospital records, x-rays and other diagnostic tools. Because the plaintiff is making the claim of negligence, that side first presents evidence. Then the defense gets its turn. If there is more than one defendant, each defendant has a turn at presenting evidence, usually in the order listed on the complaint. Each defendant presents evidence and rebuttals to the plaintiff's evidence. This provides all parties to a suit the opportunity to present a strong view of their arguments by citing supportive evidence and presenting favorable witnesses. The object of trial counsel, whether plaintiff or defense, is to undermine the credibility of the other side's case. This is the adversarial system at its best. It beats trial by combat or ordeal.

The defendant physician's role during the trial is of utmost importance. As stated elsewhere, be attentive, calm, and unemotional during all testimony. Be attentive and allow yourself to get in the flow of what is occurring in the courtroom. While trials are stressful, occasionally funny things occur and can cause a laugh during a trial. It is okay to laugh when everyone else seems to be enjoying the moment. This type of a response will allow the jury to see you as a person of good humor even in a trying situation.

We need to emphasize that a defendant should not make a lot of notes during a trial or talk to the defense attorney while he or she is listening to testimony. Your attorney must listen carefully to the questions being asked and to the way that they are answered. Your attorney will analyze each answer and its potential impact on the jury so that he or she can act on your behalf most effectively. He or she cannot listen to you and the testimony at the same time. The jury will base its verdict on the evidence presented and not on your interactions with counsel.

Keep in mind that the jury has heard the opening statements and has a fair grasp of the issues. You will be hearing detrimental things related to your care from the plaintiff's witnesses. If you were to hear only good things, you wouldn't be in court. If the jury hears a bad thing about you, you can be sure that at least one pair of eyes will look in your direction to see your response. What do you think they might conclude if they see you feverishly writing notes as bad things are being said? Because you don't know what the reaction of a juror might be, it is best not to let them make that observation. If you and your lawyer are well prepared, you will know the tone of what will be said by the plaintiff's counsel and his or her witnesses. Don't let anyone see you sweat.

The Plaintiff's Case

During the plaintiff's case, counsel for the plaintiff has the right to call you as a witness as if on cross-examination. You need to be aware that this might happen before the trial begins, and be prepared to be called in the plaintiff's case. Because you may be asked leading questions (a leading question contains the answer to the question and simply calls for a yes or no answer. For example "Your name is Dr. Smith, is that right?"), you must be well prepared for this portion of the case and feel comfortable on the stand. If you have never been in a court room, make an appointment with counsel to visit the room in which your case will be heard. Sit in the witness chair and have your attorney point out where the jury will sit and where counsel will stand during questioning. Be familiar with the surroundings and practice a few questions with counsel so that you can get a feel for the witness box.

If you are called to be cross-examined in the plaintiff's portion of the case, you may take the medical records to the stand with you if the judge grants permission. Look at the jurors when answering questions. It is the jury that is the "hearer of fact," not opposing counsel. Be congenial and courteous to counsel but be prepared to defend yourself. If asked for a yes or no answer that you want to explain in more detail, give the yes or no answer but ask the judge if you may explain the basis for your response. If allowed by the court, give the more detailed reply. If denied, your lawyer will re-ask the question during direct examination in the defense portion of the case. This will provide you the opportunity to fully explain to the jury. Do not allow opposing counsel to put you in the position of answering yes or no to every question. Find some other way to answer if you see that this is happening. For example, you might answer by saying, "Counsel, if by that question you mean, a,b,c, then my answer is yes." Answer each question truthfully and listen attentively before answering. If a yes or no answer is the only appropriate response, give it with conviction. Never let the jury see any sign of bitterness or arrogance, and *avoid* responses that are glib or sarcastic. A stupid question should be patiently answered without being patronizing. You can best protect yourself on the stand by being assertive and firm in your presentation.

Your pre-trial deposition and the medical records will be the basis on which you will be cross-examined by the plaintiff's attorney and you should be well prepared to deal with anything in the record and statements made in deposition. You can be assured that you will be challenged if your trial testimony is at all different from the statements in your deposition. If you are well prepared, variations in testimony should not occur. If faced with an obvious contradiction, acknowledge the inconsistency and explain why your answer changed. Don't panic if something that you said previously is slightly different from your current testimony. That is to be expected and can be easily handled. When you are mentally and emotionally prepared, cross-examination can be a great opportunity for you because the jury gets to hear from you during the plaintiff's case and again when your attorney examines you during the defense portion of the trial. That gives you two bites of the apple.

During the plaintiff's case presentation, the plaintiff and perhaps the spouse will testify. Their medical expert witness as well as other witnesses, such as an economist or accountant, will be called. The purpose of an economist is to reduce to present value the cost of future medical care and the value of future wages lost. You may also hear from a psychologist or psychiatrist on mental issues and from employers and fellow workers regarding lost earnings. The purpose of these witnesses is to establish the claim of malpractice and to determine the extent of monetary damages caused by the alleged negligence. Your concern is the malpractice claim, and your attention should be addressed primarily to the witnesses called on that issue. Allow your attorney and the insurance carrier to deal with the monetary issues.

When the plaintiff has rested, your attorney has the right to move that the court grant a directed verdict in your favor on one or more of the trial issues. Directed verdicts are based on the plaintiff's inability to prove its case. If granted, the trial is over. If granted, but only in part or if the motion is overruled, the defense case starts.

The Defense Case

The defense case consists of calling you, your medical expert witnesses, and other witnesses needed to establish compliance with the standard of care. Additional witnesses may include your staff and other health care professionals who have seen or treated the plaintiff. The sequential scheduling of witnesses depends, in part, on the availability of your expert witnesses. We urge that all of your witnesses appear in person to testify. Although the video testimony of expert witnesses is permissible, we feel strongly that it should be used only in very rare instances. Most experts do make arrangements to appear live. *Do not, under any circumstances, talk to any expert who will be called in your defense.* Only bad things occur when you violate this rule. The appearance of inappropriate influence on a witness is very damaging.

At some time during the defense's presentation, you will be called to the stand. This is the moment of truth for which you have prepared. You will be appropriately dressed, well rested, and ready to confidently tell the jury your side of the case. You and your attorney will be following the script on which you have agreed. The questions presented will come in logical and sequential order to provide the jury with details about your background and your role in the patient's care. Make eye contact with the jury as you answer the questions posed. It is the jury that must understand what was done and why. Answer each question truthfully and thoughtfully. Pause before answering each question and don't appear rehearsed. Be confident and assertive.

You may be asked to explain a document, an anatomy chart, an x-ray, or other study to help explain what occurred in this case. The presentation should be rehearsed with counsel prior to trial in order for you to fulfill your role as teacher to the jury. If you have had no teaching experience, take the model, chart, or other evidence home and practice your testimony with your spouse. Be open to comments about your delivery and the content of your presentation. Remember that you will be addressing a jury that doesn't understand anything about medicine, so use language that your non-medical friends would understand.

After having testified on direct examination, you will be cross-examined by the plaintiff's counsel. This will occur even if you were called as a witness during the plaintiff's case. Be confident in your attitude and demeanor. It is essential that the jury feel that you are telling the truth; do nothing to change that perception. Answer questions thoughtfully and if necessary, ask permission to explain your answers in detail. We remind you to direct your responses to the jury. Looking only at the questioner when you answer excludes the jury. If you have to turn your head from counsel to the jury to answer, sit at an angle to cut down on head movement. It's not as hard as it sounds. Picture the jury as a group of patients to whom you are speaking. Play acting helps to minimize fear.

When your testimony is completed, relax. At that point you will have done as much as possible in your defense. Your part in the case is essentially over. As you return to counsel table, do not look to counsel or others for assurances. Walk directly to the table, sit down and look at the jury. If they look your way, you want them to know that you are confident that you were not negligent in the care of the plaintiff.

Closing Argument

The closing argument to the jury is the opportunity for plaintiff and defense counsel to summarize and argue their cases to the jury. At that point you must trust counsel to deliver a strong argument on your behalf. Allow counsel to decide how to argue the case based on what he or she thinks is important. Be attentive during the closing argument and relax; there is nothing more you can do. Glance at the jury from time to time, and you will see that they are generally watching counsel with interest. *Do not react in any way* to anything said during closing arguments. After your attorney has spoken, the plaintiff's lawyer has the last opportunity to address the jury. Although this may seem unfair to you, it is permitted because of the plaintiff's substantial legal burden to prove malpractice.

Jury Instructions

The trial judge will instruct (charge) the jury on the applicable law. In some states the instructions are simple, in others complicated. The best advice during jury instructions is appearing attentive. Exactly how the jury is charged is a matter of established law, with instructions added or deleted as the evidence requires.

Deliberations and Verdicts

After the jury is instructed by the judge, it retires to the jury room. The jury is provided the trial exhibits to aid them in their deliberations. The deliberations usually take several hours so it is wise to find a place to relax. When the jury has reached its verdict, the court bailiff is notified and the parties and their counsel are assembled to hear the verdict read in open court. That is the moment at which the final outcome of the ordeal is determined. In some jurisdictions the sides have the opportunity to talk to jurors who may want to discuss their reasoning in coming to a verdict. Lawyers use verdict discussions with jurors as a learning tool. If speaking with jurors is permitted, we suggest communicating with jurors only if you prevail. Speaking to jurors if your defense failed only adds insult to injury.

Reading the Verdict

Upon informing the bailiff of the completion of deliberations, the jury returns to the court room. In most jurisdictions the judge asks the jury foreman if the jury has arrived at a verdict. At times, the foreman reads the verdict. Usually, the foreman states that they have reached a verdict, and then the verdict is given to the bailiff and the judge or the clerk of court reads the verdict.

Post-Trial Motions

In the event of an unfavorable verdict, there are several avenues available to the defense in order to salvage the result. The most common post-trial motions are for a new trial or for *judgment notwithstanding the verdict* of the jury (NOV).

A motion for a new trial requires that a specific reason for vacating the jury's verdict be submitted to the judge. Among causes submitted are that the verdict is clearly against the manifest weight of the evidence, that there was jury misconduct, that there is newly discovered evidence, or that cause of injury to the plaintiff was an accident or a surprise that could not have been avoided. These motions are generally overruled unless obvious prejudicial error occurred during trial or the jury's award to the plaintiff is so large as to numb the senses.

A motion for judgment notwithstanding the verdict asks the trial court to substitute its judgment for that of the jury and to enter final judgment to the advantage of the non-prevailing party. This motion is rarely granted and applies only to those cases where everyone, including the judge and the parties, expect a certain verdict and the jury, for its own peculiar reasons, doesn't go along with what appeared to be an open and shut case.

Appeals

In most court jurisdictions the parties to a lawsuit have the right to appeal the decision of a jury. Multiple procedural issues can be addressed on appeal. Appellate Courts work only with trial documents and do not hear witnesses. Their job is to be sure that trials are conducted fairly and according to the rules of law. The appeal process is a paper war between plaintiff and defense counsels. When an appeal is raised, it is necessary for the transcript of the evidence and the judge's charge to the jury to be submitted to the Court of Appeals. This document is the basis upon which the appeal is made. Appeals are handled by attorneys; defendants and plaintiffs are not involved. As a general rule, malpractice cases that have been tried by a jury provided appropriate instructions have little chance of being reversed on appeal. The rule of thumb is, if one is to prevail, it must be at the initial trial level.

The National Practitioner Data Bank

One of the issues of greatest concern to physicians, if he or she should lose at trial or if there is a financial claim settlement, is the placing of his or her name in the National Practitioner Data Bank (NPDB). The NPDB was a part of the Health Care Quality Improvement Act of 1986. This is the record-keeping arm of the federal Department of Health and Human Services and collects data on physicians' payments to plaintiffs and on disciplinary actions against physicians. Many physicians feel that their inclusion in the NPDB is a stigma on their good names. For that reason, the bank has become a source of fear and loathing, so it is important that the reasons for its establishment be understood.

Why the Data Bank?

The NPDB, a part of Public Law 99-660, was intended to accomplish two objectives:

- To provide immunity from liability for physicians participating in good faith peer review activities within hospitals or other licensed medical units.

- To create a central clearinghouse for information related to the professional conduct of physicians.

For many years, records of physician medical conduct, competence, and malpractice history were limited to the states. Records of disciplinary actions against a physician went only as far as state medical licensure boards. Payments made as a result of malpractice judgments were reported only if they exceeded a certain dollar base; $25,000 in some states and $10,000 in others. The information was kept confidential, and it was up to the individual states to determine how to deal with issues of medical competence.

In the 1970s and '80s, it came to the attention of many states and of Congress that a number of medical practitioners whose reputations had been severely damaged because of malpractice or unprofessional conduct in the state in which they had been practicing had merely to cross a state border to start afresh in a new state. Because the individual states had no networking arrangements for the transfer of information regarding the limitation of privileges, disciplinary actions, or medical malpractice awards, no pertinent information was passed on to the physician's new state of residence. Some of the physicians identified by state and federal investigations in the 1970s had painfully long histories of misconduct and incompetence and were practicing medicine on unsuspecting patients under the aegis of uninformed medical boards.

Title IV of P.L. 99-660 established the NPDB to provide a network system for the states to become informed about matters related to physician conduct and to provide health care institutions with a tool to screen medical staffs. It is required that hospitals and health care entities that conduct peer review investigate each physician's record in the NPDB prior to medical staff appointment and every two years thereafter.

What Information Does the Bank Collect?

Four categories of reportable data go to the NPDB. *First* are medical malpractice payments. Insurance companies and institutions must report any payments made on behalf of any licensed physician to the state's medical licensing board. That board, in turn, reports it to the NPDB. If a payment or payments are made by any of the entities indicated in the law to a plaintiff after a written complaint or claim of malpractice has been filed with a court, the payment must be reported to the NPDB; failure to do so violates both state and federal laws. If an entire settlement is made out-of pocket by the defendant physician(s) to settle a claim as the result of a legal judgment, those payments are not required to be reported to the NPDB by the law. *Second* are licensure actions taken by state medical boards. These boards must report any disciplinary actions related to professional conduct or competence to the NPDB. *Third* are any actions to limit or reduce clinical privileges taken by a hospital or other health care entity. These actions, which include denial, suspension, or revocation of any practice-related privileges, must be reported to state medical boards. Reports to state medical boards and the NPDB cannot be avoided by the voluntary surrender of the clinical privileges of a physician. *Fourth* are adverse membership actions by a professional society, such as a state or local medical association, involved in peer review. These actions must also be reported to the state licensing board and subsequently to the NPDB.

Confidentiality and the Data Bank

The information that goes into the bank, at the time of this writing, is confidential and limited to query by a limited number of entities. There are a number of consumer groups currently trying to make that information public. The groups that now have access to the information are hospitals, state licensing boards, and other health care entities with active formal peer review. Individual practitioners may review their own files by submitting an information request form, which is available from the NPDB (call 1-800-767-6732 or write to The Data Bank-P.O. Box 10832, Chantilly, VA 20153-0832 or, for overnight mail, The Data Bank 4094 Majestic Lane, PMB, Fairfax, VA. 22033, or e-mail *help@npdb-hipdb.hrsa.gov*).

Plaintiff lawyers may, under certain circumstances, also gain access to the bank's data. In the case in which hospital and physician are both sued, and it is alleged that the hospital failed to make the required query regarding the physician to the bank, attorneys may petition the Secretary of Health and Human Services for the data. Otherwise, the files are available only to the four authorized parties named above. Violation of the confidentiality of the bank can lead to fines of $10,000 for each violation, and prison terms are stipulated in the law for other violations.

If Your Name Falls into the Data Bank

It's a good idea for physicians to check their status in the bank every couple of years. One may conduct what is called, a Practitioner Self Query. Write to the addresses above or call for a request form. Mistakes do occur, and perfectly innocent names have been inadvertently placed in the file. Some hospital medical staff offices allow their licensed physicians to look at their copy of his file, but that is purely a favor and is not required of the hospital or peer review organizations.

When a practitioners' name goes into the NPDB, he should receive a Practitioner Notification Document. Upon receipt of the notice, he has 60 days to dispute the accuracy of the report. If the report is accurate, there is no issue, but, if not, he may mark and sign the Practitioner Notification Document in the "disputed status" space so that the office of the Secretary of Health and Human Services can proceed with an investigation. The specific cause of disagreement can be written on the form but there is little space to do so (60 words), so if one is to state his or her case, he or she must be concise. The entity that filed the original report should be contacted as well, and arrangements should be made to have the disagreement discussed. Sometimes the reporting entity will make a correction to its report and occasionally the report is withdrawn because of error. For further details on the process, call or write the AMA for its informational bulletin on the subject:

AMA Legal Department
515 N. State Street
Chicago, IL 60610
Telephone number: 800-262-3211

If a physician becomes involved in any of the areas of dispute that can lead to having his or her name placed in the NPDB, we recommend that an attorney with experiences in medicolegal issues be consulted. There are always risks of an unfortunate outcome in medical interventions that can cause a physician to be listed. Having one's name placed in the NPDB does not mean that the individual is a poor or incompetent physician, but it does indicate that there have been practice-related problems that require documentation. To minimize the likelihood of having a malpractice claim or a disciplinary action place ones' name in the bank, it is important to recall the four A's of medical practice — ability, affability, availability, and attentiveness — along with the big D — documentation.

The authors of this book hope that you have found it to be informative in regards to the legal issues surrounding medical practice. The avoidance of medical malpractice claims for physicians and other health care providers is our primary objective. If you have read the book carefully and follow our suggestions, you can reduce litigation exposures substantially, in your practice, hospital or other medical care environment. As you become more informed about the legal issues that surround medical practice, you will feel more able to deal with the legal system and the issues of malpractice liability in a preventive, expedient, and appropriate manner. Finally, we hope that reading this book has allayed the common concerns about dealing with liability exposures by helping you to understand the many reasonable and prudent steps that you can take to structure a medical practice well insulated from legal exposures. Being aware of the pitfalls is the first step to avoiding problems.

CPSIA information can be obtained at www.ICGtesting.com
Printed in the USA
243746LV00002B/6/P